Telehealth for Pediatricians

Editors

C. JASON WANG
JOSIP CAR
BARRY S. ZUCKERMAN

PEDIATRIC CLINICS
OF NORTH AMERICA

www.pediatric.theclinics.com

Consulting Editor
BONITA F. STANTON

August 2020 • Volume 67 • Number 4

ELSEVIER

1600 John F. Kennedy Boulevard ● Suite 1800 ● Philadelphia, Pennsylvania, 19103-2899

http://www.theclinics.com

THE PEDIATRIC CLINICS OF NORTH AMERICA Volume 67, Number 4
August 2020 ISSN 0031-3955, ISBN-13: 978-0-323-71087-9

Editor: Kerry Holland
Developmental Editor: Casey Potter

The Pediatric Clinics of North America (ISSN 0031-3955) is published bimonthly by Elsevier Inc., 360 Park Avenue South, New York, NY 10010-1710. Months of issue are February, April, June, August, October, and December. Periodicals postage paid at New York, NY and additional mailing offices. Subscription prices are $240.00 per year (US individuals), $695.00 per year (US institutions), $315.00 per year (Canadian individuals), $924.00 per year (Canadian institutions), $362.00 per year (international individuals), $924.00 per year (international institutions), $100.00 per year (US students and residents), $100.00 per year (Canadian students and residents), and $165.00 per year (international residents and students). To receive students/resident rare, orders must be accompanied by name of affiliated institution, date of term, and the signature of program/residency coordinator on institution letterhead. Orders will be billed at individual rate until proof of status is received. Foreign air speed delivery is included in all *Clinics* subscription prices. All prices are subject to change without notice. **POSTMASTER:** Send address changes to *The Pediatric Clinics of North America*, Elsevier Health Sciences Division, Subscription Customer Service, 3251 Riverport Lane, Maryland Heights, MO 63043. **Customer Service: 1-800-654-2452 (US and Canada). From outside of the US and Canada: 1-314-447-8871. Fax: 1-314-447-8029. For print support, E-mail: JournalsCustomerService-usa@elsevier.com. For online support, E-mail: JournalsOnlineSupport-usa@elsevier.com.**

Reprints. For copies of 100 or more, of articles in this publication, please contact the Commercial Reprints Department, Elsevier Inc., 360 Park Avenue South, New York, NY 10010-1710. Tel.: 212-633-3874; Fax: 212-633-3820; E-mail: reprints@elsevier.com.

The Pediatric Clinics of North America is also published in Spanish by McGraw-Hill Inter-americana Editores S.A., Mexico City, Mexico; in Portuguese by Riechmann and Affonso Editores, Rua Comandante Coelho 1085, CEP 21250, Rio de Janeiro, Brazil; and in Greek by Althayia SA, Athens, Greece.

The Pediatric Clinics of North America is covered in *MEDLINE/PubMed (Index Medicus), Excerpta Medica, Current Contents, Current Contents/Clinical Medicine, Science Citation Index, ASCA, ISI/BIOMED,* and *BIOSIS*.

PROGRAM OBJECTIVE
The goal of the *Pediatric Clinics of North America* is to keep practicing physicians and residents up to date with current clinical practice in pediatrics by providing timely articles reviewing the state-of-the-art in patient care.

TARGET AUDIENCE
All practicing pediatricians, physicians and healthcare professionals who provide patient care to pediatric patients.

LEARNING OBJECTIVES
Upon completion of this activity, participants will be able to:
1. Review the implementation of telehealth by utilizing various delivery methods such as asynchronously, synchronously, and/or remotely within select patient populations and practice settings.
2. Discuss successful strategies for the adoption and expansion of telehealth including privacy and security measures, current state and federal policies, and the lack of cost-benefit analyses.
3. Recognize the benefits of communication, counseling, and remote patient monitoring associated with the implementation of telehealth within select patient populations and practice settings.

ACCREDITATIONS
Physician Credit

The Elsevier Office of Continuing Medical Education (EOCME) is accredited by the Accreditation Council for Continuing Medical Education (ACCME) to provide continuing medical education for physicians.

The EOCME designates this journal-based activity(s) for a maximum of 17 *AMA PRA Category 1 Credit*(s)™. Physicians should claim only the credit commensurate with the extent of their participation in the activity.

All other healthcare professionals requesting continuing education credit for this this journal-based activity will be issued a certificate of participation.

ABP Maintenance of Certification Credit

Successful completion of this CME activity, which includes participation in the activity and individual assessment of and feedback to the learner, enables the learner to earn up to 17 MOC points in the American Board of Pediatrics' (ABP) Maintenance of Certification (MOC) program. It is the CME activity provider's responsibility to submit learner completion information to ACCME for the purpose of granting ABP MOC credit.

DISCLOSURE OF CONFLICTS OF INTEREST
The EOCME assesses conflict of interest with its instructors, faculty, planners, and other individuals who are in a position to control the content of CME activities. All relevant conflicts of interest that are identified are thoroughly vetted by EOCME for fair balance, scientific objectivity, and patient care recommendations. EOCME is committed to providing its learners with CME activities that promote improvements or quality in healthcare and not a specific proprietary business or a commercial interest.

The planning committee, staff, authors and editors listed below have identified no financial relationships or relationships to products or devices they or their spouse/life partner have with commercial interest related to the content of this CME activity:

Manuel C. Alvarado, BS; Alejandra Barrero-Castillero, MD, MPH; Matthew F. Bouchonville, MD; Eli M. Cahan, BBA; Cristina Camayd-Muñoz, MS; Josip Car, MD, PhD; Angela C. Chen, BS; Ng Kee Chong, MBBS, MMed (Paeds), FAMS; Brian K. Corwin, MD; Victor Cueto, MD, MS; Nicolas Cuttriss, MD, MPH; Jillian Orr Daglilar, EdM; Dirk F. de Korne, PhD, MSc; Laurie M. Douglass, MD; Chew Chu Shan Elaine, MBBS, M Med(Paeds), MRCPCh (UK), MCI; Laura Fisher; Jennifer L. Fogel, PhD; Sashikumar Ganapathy, Mb Bch Bao(NUI), MRCPCH(UK), MHPE(Maastrict); Kerry Holland; Julianna C. Hsing, BA; Rinat R. Jonas, MD; Marilu Kelly, MSN, RN, CNE, CHCP; Tzielan Lee, MD; Tiffany T. Liu; Elaine Lum, MClinPharm, PhD; Jasmin Ma, BS; David M. Maahs, MD, PhD; Callie A. Margiotta, BS; Rajkumar Mayakrishnan, BSc, MBA; Vandna Mittal, MPH; Chun Y. Ng, MBA, MPH; Madeline H. Niemann, BA; Tamara T. Perry, MD; Rajdeep Pooni, MD; Jennifer K. Raymond, MD, MCR; Christy Sandborg, MD; Lee M. Sanders, MD, MPH; Nirav R. Shah, MD, MPH; Sonoo Thadaney-Israni, MBA; Elif Seda Selamet Tierney, MD; Louise Sandra van Galen, MD, PhD; Deborah K. Vanderveen, MD; Ashby F. Walker, PhD; C. Jason Wang, MD, PhD; Jodi K. Wenger, MD; Paul H. Wise, MD, MPH; Phoebe H. Yager, MD; Barry Zuckerman, MD.

UNAPPROVED/OFF-LABEL USE DISCLOSURE

The EOCME requires CME faculty to disclose to the participants:

1. When products or procedures being discussed are off-label, unlabelled, experimental, and/or investigational (not US Food and Drug Administration [FDA] approved); and
2. Any limitations on the information presented, such as data that are preliminary or that represent ongoing research, interim analyses, and/or unsupported opinions. Faculty may discuss information about pharmaceutical agents that is outside of FDA-approved labelling. This information is intended solely for CME and is not intended to promote off-label use of these medications. If you have any questions, contact the medical affairs department of the manufacturer for the most recent prescribing information.

TO ENROLL

To enroll in the *Pediatric Clinics of North America* Continuing Medical Education program, call customer service at 1-800-654-2452 or sign up online at http://www.theclinics.com/home/cme. The CME program is available to subscribers for an additional annual fee of USD 300.00.

METHOD OF PARTICIPATION

In order to claim credit, participants must complete the following:

1. Complete enrolment as indicated above.
2. Read the activity.
3. Complete the CME Test and Evaluation. Participants must achieve a score of 70% on the test. All CME Tests and Evaluations must be completed online.

In order to claim MOC points, participants must complete the following:

1. Complete steps listed above for claiming CME credit
2. Provide your specialty board ID#, birth date (MM/DD), and attestation.
3. Online MOC submission is only available for the American Board of pediatrics' (ABP) Maintenance of Certification (MOC) program

CME INQUIRIES/SPECIAL NEEDS

For all CME inquiries or special needs, please contact elsevierCME@elsevier.com.

Contributors

CONSULTING EDITOR

BONITA F. STANTON, MD
Founding Dean, Hackensack Meridian School of Medicine at Seton Hall University, President, Academic Enterprise, Hackensack Meridian Health Robert C. and Laura C. Garrett Endowed Chair for the School of Medicine, Professor of Pediatrics, Nutley, New Jersey, USA

EDITORS

C. JASON WANG, MD, PhD
Director, Center for Policy, Outcomes, and Prevention, Associate Professor of Pediatrics (General Pediatrics), Medicine (Primary Care Outcomes Research), and Health Research and Policy, Co-Chair, Mobile Health and Other New Technologies, Center for Population Health Sciences, Stanford School of Medicine, Stanford, California, USA

JOSIP CAR, MD, PhD, DIC, MSc, FFPH, FRCP (Edin)
Associate Professor of Health Services Outcomes Research, Director, Health Services Outcomes Research Programme, Director, Centre for Population Health Sciences, Principal Investigator, Population Health & Living Laboratory, Centre for Population Health Sciences, Lee Kong Chian School of Medicine, Nanyang Technological University, Singapore, Singapore

BARRY S. ZUCKERMAN, MD
Professor and Chair Emeritus, Department of Pediatrics, Boston University School of Medicine, Boston, Massachusetts, USA

AUTHORS

MANUEL C. ALVARADO, BS
Division of Pediatric Neurology, Boston Medical Center, MPH Candidate, Class of 2020, Boston University School of Public Health, Boston, Massachusetts, USA

ALEJANDRA BARRERO-CASTILLERO, MD, MPH
Division of Neonatology, Beth Israel Deaconess Medical Center, Division of Newborn Medicine, Boston Children's Hospital, Boston, Massachusetts, USA

MATTHEW F. BOUCHONVILLE, MD
Associate Professor, Division of Endocrinology, Diabetes, Medical Director, Endo ECHO, University of New Mexico School of Medicine Albuquerque, New Mexico, USA

ELI M. CAHAN, BBA
Clinical Excellence Research Center, Stanford School of Medicine, Stanford, California, USA; NYU Grossman School of Medicine, New York, New York, USA

CRISTINA CAMAYD-MUÑOZ, MS
Project Manager, Division of Pediatric Neurology, Boston, Massachusetts, USA

JOSIP CAR, MD, PhD, DIC, MSc, FFPH, FRCP (Edin)
Associate Professor of Health Services Outcomes Research, Director, Health Services Outcomes Research Programme, Director, Centre for Population Health Sciences, Principal Investigator, Population Health & Living Laboratory, Centre for Population Health Sciences, Lee Kong Chian School of Medicine, Nanyang Technological University, Singapore, Singapore

ANGELA C. CHEN, BS
Division of Pediatric Cardiology, Department of Pediatrics, Stanford University Medical Center, Palo Alto, California, USA

CHEW CHU SHAN ELAINE, MBBS, MMed(Paeds), MRCPCh (UK), MCI
Consultant, Adolescent Medicine Service, Department of Paediatrics, KK Women's & Children's Hospital, Singapore, Singapore

BRIAN K. CORWIN, MD
Department of Radiology, Cleveland Clinic Foundation, Imaging Institute, Cleveland, Ohio, USA

VICTOR CUETO, MD, MS
Division of General Internal Medicine, Department Internal Medicine, Assistant Professor, Rutgers New Jersey Medical School, Newark, New Jersey, USA

NICOLAS CUTTRISS, MD, MPH
Clinical Assistant Professor, Director Project ECHO Diabetes, Division of Endocrinology, Department of Pediatrics, Stanford School of Medicine, Stanford, California, USA

JILLIAN ORR DAGLILAR, EdM
Executive Producer, WGBH Educational Foundation, Columbia, Missouri, USA

DIRK F. DE KORNE, PhD, MSc, Duke-NUS School of Medicine, Deputy Director, Medical Innovation & Care Transformation, KK Women's & Children's Hospital, Singapore, Singapore; Adjunct Assistant Professor, Erasmus School of Health Policy and Management, Erasmus University Rotterdam, Rotterdam, Netherlands; Director, Care & Welfare, SVRZ Cares in Zeeland, Middelburg, SVRZ, Middelburg, Netherlands

LAURIE M. DOUGLASS, MD
Associate Professor of Pediatrics and Neurology, Division of Pediatric Neurology, Boston Medical Center, Boston, Massachusetts, USA

JENNIFER L. FOGEL, PhD
Division of Endocrinology, Department of Pediatrics, Children's Hospital Los Angeles, Los Angeles, California, USA

SASHIKUMAR GANAPATHY, MB BCh Bao, MRCPCH(UK), MSc
Adjunct Assistant Professor, Emergency Medicine, KK Women's & Children's Hospital, Duke-NUS School of Medicine, Singapore, Singapore

JULIANNA C. HSING, BA
Master of Science Candidate, Department of Epidemiology and Population Health, Stanford School of Medicine, Stanford, California, USA

RINAT R. JONAS, MD
Assistant Professor of Pediatrics and Neurology, Division of Pediatric Neurology, Boston Medical Center, Boston, Massachusetts, USA

TZIELAN LEE, MD
Clinical Associate Professor of Pediatrics, Rheumatology, Lucile Packard Children's Hospital, Stanford, California, USA

TIFFANY T. LIU
Research Intern, Center for Policy, Outcomes and Prevention, Stanford School of Medicine, Stanford, California, USA

ELAINE LUM, MClinPharm, PhD
Senior Research Fellow, Digital Health, Centre for Population Health Sciences, Lee Kong Chian School of Medicine, Nanyang Technological University, Singapore, Singapore; Visiting Clinical Fellow, School of Clinical Sciences, Faculty of Health, Queensland University of Technology, Australia

DAVID M. MAAHS, MD, PhD
Professor of Pediatrics and, by courtesy, of Health Research and Policy (Epidemiology), Chief of Pediatric Endocrinology, Lucile Packard Children's Hospital, Associate Director, Stanford Diabetes Research Center, Division of Endocrinology, Department of Pediatrics, Stanford School of Medicine, Stanford, California, USA

CALLIE A. MARGIOTTA, BS
Arkansas Children's Research Institute, Little Rock, Arkansas, USA

VANDNA MITTAL, MPH
Stanford Children's Health, Stanford, California, USA

CHUN Y. NG, MBA, MPH
Project Manager, New School for Leadership in Healthcare, Koo Foundation Sun Yat-Sen Cancer, Taipei, Taiwan

NG KEE CHONG, MBBS, MMed(Paeds), FAMS (Singapore), FRCPCH (UK), eMBA
Senior Consultant, Medical Innovation & Care Transformation, Division of Medicine, KK Women's & Children's Hospital, Duke-NUS School of Medicine, Singapore, Singapore

MADELINE H. NIEMANN, BA
Research Assistant, Division of Pediatric Neurology, Boston Medical Center, Boston, Massachusetts, USA

TAMARA T. PERRY, MD
Department of Pediatrics, University of Arkansas for Medical Sciences, Arkansas Children's Research Institute, Little Rock, Arkansas, USA

RAJDEEP POONI, MD
Clinical Fellow, Pediatric Rheumatology, Lucile Packard Children's Hospital, Stanford, California, USA

JENNIFER K. RAYMOND, MD, MCR
Division of Endocrinology, Department of Pediatrics, Children's Hospital Los Angeles, Associate Professor of Clinical Pediatrics, Keck School of Medicine of the University of Southern California, Los Angeles, California, USA

CHRISTY SANDBORG, MD
Professor of Pediatrics, Rheumatology, Lucile Packard Children's Hospital, Stanford, California, USA

LEE M. SANDERS, MD, MPH
Division of General Pediatrics, Department of Pediatrics, Associate Professor of Pediatrics, Division Chief, Stanford School of Medicine, Stanford, California, USA

ELIF SEDA SELAMET TIERNEY, MD
Associate Professor of Pediatrics, Division of Pediatric Cardiology, Department of Pediatrics, Stanford University Medical Center, Palo Alto, California, USA

NIRAV R. SHAH, MD, MPH
Clinical Excellence Research Center, Stanford School of Medicine, Stanford, California, USA

SONOO THADANEY-ISRANI, MBA
Department of Medicine, Stanford School of Medicine, Stanford, California, USA

LOUISE SANDRA VAN GALEN, MD, PhD
Research Fellow, Acute Internal Medicine, Department of Internal Medicine, Amsterdam University Medical Center, Location VUmc, Amsterdam, Netherlands

DEBORAH K. VANDERVEEN, MD
Department of Ophthalmology, Boston Children's Hospital, Boston, Massachusetts, USA

ASHBY F. WALKER, PhD
Assistant Professor, Health Services Research, Management, and Policy, Director for Health Equity Initiatives, University of Florida Diabetes Institute, Project Director, ECHO Diabetes Florida, University of Florida, Gainesville, Florida, USA

C. JASON WANG, MD, PhD
Director, Center for Policy, Outcomes, and Prevention, Associate Professor of Pediatrics (General Pediatrics), Medicine (Primary Care Outcomes Research), and Health Research and Policy, Co-Chair, Mobile Health and Other New Technologies, Center for Population Health Sciences, Stanford School of Medicine, Stanford, California, USA

JODI K. WENGER, MD
Division of Pediatric Neurology, Pediatrician, Division of Pediatrics, Boston Medical Center, Boston, Massachusetts, USA

PAUL H. WISE, MD, MPH
Richard E. Behrman Professor in Child Health and Society, Professor, Department of Pediatrics, Stanford School of Medicine, Stanford, California, USA

PHOEBE H. YAGER, MD
Assistant Professor, Harvard Medical School, Massachusetts General Hospital, Boston, Massachusetts, USA

BARRY ZUCKERMAN, MD
Professor and Chair Emeritus, Department of Pediatrics, Boston University School of Medicine, Boston, Massachusetts, USA

Contents

Section I: Overview

Telehealth can be delivered asynchronously, synchronously, or through remote patient monitoring. The cost of telehealth, patient use, and effectiveness vary by the technology deployed and by specialty. Telehealth use requires patient and provider adaptability. The improvement of telehealth is restricted by state and federal policies as well as privacy and security concerns. Current telehealth literature provides more consistent evidence of benefits for communication and counseling, and from remote patient monitoring of chronic conditions. However, the benefits and costs of telehealth programs are highly dependent on the technology used, the medical condition studied, and the health care context.

This article focuses on the role of text messaging and messaging applications, discusses technical and legal issues, and reviews current examples of the application of text messaging in the clinical adult and pediatric practice. Reviews of current examples of text messaging in adult and pediatric practice show uptake has been increasing substantially in recent years. In pediatric care text messaging has been used for behavior intervention and outcomes tracking. Although applications are promising, the potential of nonsynchronic messaging in the formal delivery of care is still in the neonatal phase compared with its grown-up existence in day-to-day modern life.

Section II: The Nuts and Bolts of How to Implement Telehealth: Examples from Different Pediatric Specialties and Subspecialties

Pediatric patients with uncontrolled asthma often live in underserved areas such as rural communities where few pediatric asthma specialists exist. There are significant costs associated with acute asthma exacerbations, which are increasingly prevalent in these high-risk populations. Telemedicine is a viable option when addressing barriers in access to care and cost-efficiency. Implementing telemedicine in schools and other local community settings, as well as implementing innovative technology such as smartphone applications, can reduce the burden of asthma; increase patient satisfaction; and, most importantly, improve pediatric asthma outcomes.

A team of providers, researchers, patients, and families created a novel telehealth tool to improve communication across a variety of systems involved in pediatric epilepsy care. This tool facilitates in-home telemedicine appointments and saves costs for patients and hospital systems alike within the context of a population highly affected by health care disparities.

Telehealth is a promising new tool in medicine that has changed the landscape of medical care. The benefits of telehealth technology are immense, including improved access to care and potential savings in monetary and opportunity costs. Current challenges of incorporating telehealth services into regular clinical care include licensure and regulatory barriers, difficulty obtaining insurance reimbursements, and high costs of setting up successful telehealth infrastructures. These challenges threaten telehealth's future scalability and expansion to reach all patients in need.

This article describes the present state of telemedicine in pediatric rheumatology. Specifically, it addresses the potential use of telemedicine to increase patient-provider access as well as its potential clinical limitations. The work also briefly describes the next steps with respect to telemedicine research as well as some new research findings specifically for pediatric rheumatology.

Telehealth is well positioned to address the common challenges of providing high-quality care to children and adolescents with obesity. The potential benefits of telehealth for pediatric obesity are applicable across the full spectrum of care from diagnosis and assessment to ongoing management. This article reviews the emerging field of telehealth for the treatment of pediatric obesity. The challenges of the current approach to pediatric obesity care are explored, and the potential benefits of incorporating and implementing telehealth in this field are presented. The care of pediatric patients with obesity is particularly well suited for telehealth.

Although most pediatric intensive care units invite parents to participate in daily rounds, many families face barriers preventing them from being physically present on rounds. Telehealth for remote parent participation on daily rounds offers one solution to this problem. However, barriers threaten the implementation and sustainability of such programs. Highly reliable, user-friendly telehealth technologies coupled with adequate human resources to address logistical challenges and clinical champions to affect culture change are key. Further research is needed to better quantify the impact of such programs on patient and parent outcomes and to convince hospital leadership to invest in telehealth solutions.

Management of type 1 diabetes mellitus for pediatric and young adult patients is well suited for telehealth. Diabetes management requires frequent communication with health care providers as well as the interpretation of many types of data that can be measured in the home and shared virtually to the provider by the patient. Telehealth technologies allow for a safe alternative and/or addition to in-person care for youth with diabetes. Telehealth increases access to health care, saves time and money, and results in improvements in rates of appointment adherence, patient satisfaction, and quality of life.

Age-specific recommendations contain extensive information that cannot be presented adequately in pediatric preventative care visits. Parental guidance is important, especially for children with social and/or medical risks, but existing evidence-based interventions tend to be resource intensive and difficult to scale. Because the use of mobile technology is now prevalent even among low-income families, the benefits of utilizing the Internet and mobile apps to improve parental guidance are active areas of research. Analyses of patient-generated data from mobile apps may help identify effective ways to use social influences, social learning, and social networks for improving population health.

Section III: Issues Related to the Adoption, Implementation, Scalability, Sustainability, and Adherence of Health Apps and Telemedicine Programs

Telehealth and telemedicine services can be a solution for improving accessibility and reducing the cost of health care. Challenges remain in designing, implementing, and sustainably scaling telehealth solutions. Research is lacking on the health impacts and cost-effectiveness of telehealth; more data are needed in the evaluation of telehealth programs, adjusting for potential participant bias and extending the time frame of evaluating impact. In addition, rethinking and addressing the economic incentives and payment for telehealth services, as well as the medical-legal framework for provider competition across geographic regions (and jurisdictions), are needed for greater adoption of telehealth services.

Pediatric practice increasingly involves providing care for children with medical complexity. Telehealth offers a strategy for providers and health care systems to improve care for these patients and their families. However, lack of awareness related to the unintended negative consequences of telehealth on vulnerable populations–coupled with failure to intentional design best practices for telehealth initiatives–implies that these novel technologies may worsen health disparities in the long run. This article reviews the positive and negative implications of telehealth. In addition, to achieve optimal implementation of telehealth, it discusses 10 considerations to promote optimal care of children using these technologies.

This article explores the impact of digital technologies, including telehealth, teleconsultations, wireless devices, and chatbots, in pediatrics. Automated digital health with the Internet of things will allow better collection of real-world data for generation of real-world evidence to improve child health. Artificial intelligence with predictive analytics in turn will drive evidence-based decision-support systems and deliver personalized care to children. This technology creates building blocks for a learning child health and health care ecosystem.

Section IV: Telehealth Training and Tele-education

Retinopathy of prematurity (ROP) is the leading cause of childhood blindness in very-low-birthweight and very preterm infants in the United States. With improved survival of smaller babies, more infants are at risk for ROP, yet there is an increasing shortage of providers to screen and treat ROP. Through a literature review of new and emerging technologies, screening criteria, and analysis of a national survey of pediatric ophthalmologists and retinal specialists, the authors found the shortage of ophthalmology workforce for ROP a serious and growing concern. When used appropriately, emerging technologies have the potential to mitigate gaps in the ROP workforce.

Doctors need to acquire telehealth consultation skills to thrive in the increasingly pressurized health system of delivering high-quality, high-volume health care with a shrinking health care workforce. Telehealth consultations require the same degree of thoroughness and careful clinical judgment as face-to-face consultations. The distinct differences between telehealth and face-to-face consultations warrant training in telehealth, which should be incorporated into core curricula of medical schools and continuing medical education. We describe competency-based training for telehealth piloted with medical residents. The use of competency-based training for telehealth operationalized as an entrustable professional activity will facilitate high-quality, safe, and effective telehealth consultations.

Lack of access to subspecialty care and persistent suboptimal outcomes for insulin-requiring patients with diabetes mandates development of innovative health care delivery models. The workforce shortage of endocrinologists in the United States results in primary care providers taking on the role of diabetes specialists despite lack of confidence and knowledge in complex diabetes management. The telementoring model Project ECHO amplifies and democratizes specialty knowledge to reduce disparities in care and improve health outcomes. Project ECHO can be applied to type 1 diabetes and other complex medical conditions to address health disparities and urgent needs of complex patients throughout the lifespan.

Telehealth has improved delivery of health care worldwide by improving access to and the quality of health care and by improving the global shortage of health professionals through collaboration and training. Although many telehealth efforts have been reported in adult health care settings, it is important to examine telehealth efforts in the pediatric setting. Children who are most commonly ill and malnourished are often those of underserved populations of the developing world. This article examines current uses of pediatric telehealth in a global setting and discusses key approaches to how telehealth may become successfully integrated and scaled in those settings.

PEDIATRIC CLINICS OF NORTH AMERICA

SERIES OF RELATED INTEREST

Clinics in Perinatology
http://www.perinatology.theclinics.com/
Advances in Pediatrics
http://www.advancesinpediatrics.com/

THE CLINICS ARE AVAILABLE ONLINE!
Access your subscription at:
www.theclinics.com

Foreword

The Era of Telehealth Has Arrived

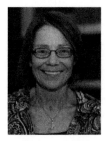

Bonita F. Stanton, MD
Consulting Editor

In planning for the next few years of publications of *Pediatric Clinics of North America*, I typically approach a potential guest editor for a topic-specific issue approximately 24 months before its anticipated publication date.

At the time I approached the guest editor (which became guest editors) for the current issue regarding telehealth or other health care innovations, I had assumed that the issue would need to include at least 2 or 3 "sets" of innovations rather than simply one (telehealth). I was concerned that the field of telehealth might be too underdeveloped and its future too uncertain to fill a complete issue. However, the guest editors for the issue assured me that with the rapid pace of development of the field, my worries would not be sustained. Even during this early developmental phase of telehealth 2 to 3 years ago, the advantages to patient, family, provider, and health system were beginning to be appreciated, including patient and physician convenience, closer follow-up, patient satisfaction, and, in some cases, cost savings. However, much work still needed to be done; publications also noted the need for greater experience, the inability to access standard technologies present only in offices or hospitals, the significance of not being able to perform a physical exam, and so forth.[1,2] The advantages of telehealth in rural areas with limited access were rapidly being appreciated[3] as was its utility in urgent care settings, offsetting any concerns.[4] In summary, I ultimately agreed that "someday" there would be a substantial role for telehealth, that this developmental phase of telehealth would make substantial progress over the next few years, and that, therefore, we could devote a full issue of *Pediatric Clinics of North America* to this important topic.

Indeed, the 17 articles in this issue provide tremendous insight into the emerging field of pediatric telehealth—and indeed in the broader field of telehealth in general. In the first 2 sections, the authors examine telehealth from a public health perspective as well as a clinical perspective, including that of specific subspecialties. These articles are important and informative for all pediatricians and childcare providers.

Pediatr Clin N Am 67 (2020) xv–xvi
https://doi.org/10.1016/j.pcl.2020.05.002
0031-3955/20/© 2020 Published by Elsevier Inc.

The last 2 sections of the issue (*Section 3: Issues Related To The Adoption, Implementation, Scalability, Sustainability* and *Adherence Over Time of Health Apps And Telemedicine Programs* and *Section 4: Telehealth Training and Tele-Education*) are especially relevant for child health care providers without prior experience with telehealth as well as for those health care providers with administrative roles determining the position that telehealth will assume in their enterprise and those with teaching roles.

But then, things changed—substantially. Most significantly—and certainly not anticipated 2 years ago—is the timing of the publication of this issue. Never in my experience with *Pediatric Clinics of North America* has an issue been published that is more timely. Since the first known case of COVID-19 arriving in the United States on January 20, 2020 (3 months ago), the use and appreciation of telehealth have exploded. The opening paragraph of *The Lancet*'s April 11, 2020 *World Report* (page 1180) states:

In the face of a surge in cases of coronavirus disease 2019 (COVID-19), physicians and health systems worldwide are racing to adopt virtualized treatment approaches that obviate the need for physical meetings between patients and health providers. But many doctors are watching warily.[5]

The article suggests that in the United States as many as half of all consultations are now being conducted through telehealth. The author suggests that among the many reasons this transition may be happening so quickly—over a matter of just 3 months—is the fact that both patients and doctors may be at risk through a face-to-face visit. But, whatever the reason, the release of this issue of *Pediatric Clinics of North America* is certainly timely.

Bonita F. Stanton, MD
Hackensack Meridian School of Medicine
at Seton Hall University
340 Kingsland Street, Building 123
Nutley, NJ 07110, USA

E-mail address:
bonita.stanton@shu.edu

REFERENCES

1. Wechsler LR. Advantages and limitations of teleneurology. JAMA Neurol 2015; 72(3):349–54.
2. Girerd N, Seronde MF, Coiro S, et al, INI-CRCT, Great Network, and the EF-HF Group. Integrative assessment of congestion in heart failure throughout the patient journey. JACC Heart Fail 2018;6(4):273–85.
3. Galea MD. Telemedicine in rehabilitation. Phys Med Rehabil Clin N Am 2019;30(2): 473–83.
4. Wilson L. Urgent care embraces telehealth. More centers see advantages of virtual services. Health Data Manag 2017;25(2):38–40.
5. Webster P. Virtual healthcare in the era of COVID-19. Lancet 2020;1180–1.

Preface

The Power of Telehealth Has Been Unleashed

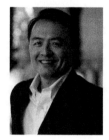
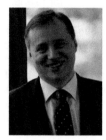
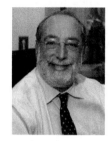

| C. Jason Wang, MD, PhD | Josip Car, MD, PhD, DIC, MSc, FFPH, FRCP (Edin) | Barry S. Zuckerman, MD |

Editors

Since the authors submitted their articles for this special issue of *Pediatric Clinics of North America* devoted to Telehealth for Pediatricians, the world has changed. The human race has been attacked by the most serious viral pandemic of our generation, the novel coronavirus disease 2019 (COVID-19). COVID-19 posed an unprecedented challenge to health delivery systems everywhere. As face-to-face clinic visits are no longer desirable due to the risk of catching the virus, COVID-19 has inadvertently aided the adoption of telehealth. The US Coronavirus Aid, Relief, and Economic Security Act passed by the US Congress has provisions to provide health care resources needed to fight COVID-19.[1] On April 23, the US Centers for Medicare and Medicaid Services (CMS) also released a tool kit for states to accelerate the adoption of telehealth in its Medicaid and Child Health Insurance Programs. The tool kit can facilitate the identification of barriers to deployment in areas such as populations eligible for telehealth, coverage and reimbursement policies, providers and practitioners eligible to provide telehealth, technology requirements, and pediatric considerations.[2]

In addition, CMS and the federal government have relaxed many previous restrictions on the use of telemedicine for Medicare to allow physicians to utilize telehealth during the COVID-19 pandemic.[1] Among them are key changes to Medicare telehealth payment policies to allow the same rate as in-office visits for all diagnoses; reduction or waiver of cost-sharing for telehealth visits and remote monitoring services, as well as code selection based on physician time spent on the date of visit or on medical decision making. Medicare also expanded access to telehealth to allow all settings (eg, home); both new and established patients; and consent for services at any time and has removed frequency limitations of Medicare telehealth services. Physicians can provide services from their homes; physicians licensed from 1 state can provide services in another state, but state licensure laws still apply. States also now have broader

Pediatr Clin N Am 67 (2020) xvii–xviii
https://doi.org/10.1016/j.pcl.2020.05.001
0031-3955/20/© 2020 Published by Elsevier Inc.

flexibility to use telehealth, such as telecommunications technology commonly available on smart phones (FaceTime, Skype, Zoom, and so forth), telephones, or remote patient monitoring; however, Facebook Live, Twitch, and TikTok or other public facing services are not acceptable to the Office of Civil Rights for HIPAA considerations. Ancillary health professionals, such as social workers, clinical psychologists, physical therapists, occupational therapists, and speech-language pathologists, will have expanded access to telehealth during the crisis. For rural health clinics and federally qualified health centers, CMS will pay $92 for telehealth provided by physicians and other practitioners.

Given that the power of telehealth has been unleashed during the COVID-19 crisis, and over half of all visits during this period are likely to be telehealth services, health systems around the world may face the next dilemma: Would patients go back to the inefficient health care delivery systems they had before, where it often involves long journeys, including parking and waiting times, to the doctor's physical offices? In this issue, authors write about policy perspectives and clinical experiences related to telehealth. It is hoped their ideas and experiences will serve as a framework for the future.

C. Jason Wang, MD, PhD
Center for Policy, Outcomes and Prevention
Stanford University School of Medicine
117 Encina Commons
Stanford, CA 94305, USA

Josip Car, MD, PhD, DIC, MSc, FFPH, FRCP (Edin)
Centre for Population Health Sciences
Lee Kong Chian School of Medicine
Nanyang Technological University
Singapore
Clinical Sciences Building
11 Mandalay Road
Singapore 308232, Singapore

Barry S. Zuckerman, MD
Department of Pediatrics
Boston University School of Medicine
72 East Concord Street
Boston, MA 02118, USA

E-mail addresses:
cjwang1@stanford.edu (C.J. Wang)
josip.car@ntu.edu.sg (J. Car)
barry.zuckerman@bmc.org (B.S. Zuckerman)

REFERENCES

1. CARES Act: AMA COVID-19 pandemic telehealth fact sheet. 2020. Available at: https://www.ama-assn.org/delivering-care/public-health/cares-act-ama-covid-19-pandemic-telehealth-fact-sheet. Accessed May 6, 2020.
2. CMS: State Medicaid & CHIP Telehealth Toolkit. 2020. Available at: https://www.medicaid.gov/medicaid/benefits/downloads/medicaid-chip-telehealth-toolkit.pdf. Accessed May 6, 2020.

The Opportunities for Telehealth in Pediatric Practice and Public Health

C. Jason Wang, MD, PhD[a],*, Jasmin Ma, BS[b,1],
Barry Zuckerman, MD[c], Josip Car, MD, PhD[d,e,2]

KEYWORDS

- Telehealth • Telemedicine • Public health • Pediatrics • Applications • Limitations
- Review

KEY POINTS

- Telehealth can be delivered asynchronously, synchronously, or through remote patient monitoring. Terms related to telehealth include digital health, connected health, telemedicine, eHealth, and mobile health.
- The cost, use, and effectiveness of telehealth vary depending on the technology deployed and by specialty.
- Telehealth use requires patient and provider adaptability, and is driven by convenience, accessibility, and increased health services demand caused by longer life-expectancies and lower mortality.
- The adoption and expansion of telehealth are restricted by current state and federal policies, privacy and security concerns, and the lack of cost-benefit analyses.
- Current telehealth literature provides more consistent evidence of benefits for communication and counseling, and from remote patient monitoring of chronic conditions. However, research is still lacking, especially in cost analyses, and is often limited by study implementations.

[a] Center for Policy, Outcomes, and Prevention, Stanford University School of Medicine, 117 Encina Commons, Stanford, CA 94305, USA; [b] Center for Policy, Outcomes and Prevention, Stanford University School of Medicine, Stanford, CA, USA; [c] Department of Pediatrics, Boston University School of Medicine, 801 Harrison Avenue, Boston, MA 02118, USA; [d] Department of Primary Care and Public Health, Imperial College London, London, UK; [e] Centre for Population Health Sciences, Lee Kong Chian School of Medicine, Nanyang Technological University, Singapore, Clinical Sciences Building, 11 Mandalay Road, Singapore 308232, Singapore
[1] Present address: 117 Encina Commons, StanfordCA 94305.
[2] Present address: Clinical Sciences Building, 11 Mandalay Road, Singapore 308232.
* Corresponding author. 117 Encina Commons, Stanford CA 94305.
E-mail address: cjwang1@stanford.edu

Pediatr Clin N Am 67 (2020) 603–611
https://doi.org/10.1016/j.pcl.2020.03.001
0031-3955/20/© 2020 Elsevier Inc. All rights reserved.

pediatric.theclinics.com

INTRODUCTION

The US Department of Health and Human Services defines telehealth as "the use of electronic information and telecommunication technologies to support and promote long-distance clinical health care, patient and professional health-related education, public health, and health administration."[1] Digital health and connected health are broad terms that refer to the use of technology to access or to integrate health services.[2–4] Related terms that are often used in conjunction include telemedicine, a subset of telehealth that refers to the delivery of clinical health care at a distance[5]; eHealth, the delivery of health services using the Internet and related technologies[6]; and mobile health, the delivery of health services using mobile devices[5] (**Fig. 1**).

USES OF TELEHEALTH

Telehealth can be delivered asynchronously via store and forward communications to transmit patient data and remote assessments; synchronously using real-time audio and video consultation, known as virtual visits; and through remote patient monitoring (RPM) using sensors and monitoring devices.[7,8]

Asynchronous Applications

Asynchronous applications increase accessibility to specialist evaluations independent of time and location. Their use includes gap service coverage, such as nighttime radiology coverage.[5] Radiologic and retinal imaging can be read by radiologists and ophthalmologists remotely and delivered to the patient's primary care provider.[3] Teledermatology is another increasingly common asynchronous

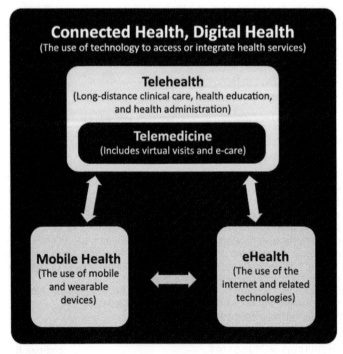

Fig. 1. The relationships between common terms associated with telehealth.

application where diagnoses are often made based on photos taken and uploaded from a patient's phone.[3] In pediatrics, common asynchronous applications include tele-echocardiography, teledermatology, and teleretinal screening.[9]

Synchronous Applications

Virtual visits have made health care more accessible generally and address some barriers for rural or underserved patients, who account for 20% of the United States' population according to the 2010 Census.[9,10] The use of scheduled virtual visits varies by specialty and includes routine follow-up, chronic condition management, medication updates, engagement of families in outpatient care, surgical preadmission testing, postoperative pain management, and postoperative follow-up.[11] Telehealth is also applicable in the improvement of coordination of care. For example, virtual visits can be used by children with chronic kidney disease for ongoing assessment of pre-transplant or established dialysis patients.[12]

Many emergency departments, urgent care centers, and intensive care units (ICUs) use virtual visits and large video consultations to improve the outcomes of acute or time-sensitive interventions (eg, stroke). Virtual visits also facilitate mandated services, such as the provision of health care to prison inmates.[5,7] Telehealth has improved outcomes in trauma incidents by allowing faster intervention during the critical period after a traumatic event.[7] For psychotherapy intervention and chronic disease management, a systematic review of 17 studies showed that the outcomes of videoconferencing groups are similar to those of in-person support groups. Thus, videoconferencing support groups may help overcome accessibility barriers such as mobility or distance.[13]

From a systematic review of pediatric telehealth, physicians made significantly fewer errors for patients who received a video consult compared with those who received a telephone consult or did not receive a consult at all. Physical examinations of neonatal ICU (NICU) patients performed and compared between on-site and off-site neonatologists showed good or excellent agreement for most assessments.[14]

Emergent new technologies

Robotic telepresence is a technology that allows face-to-face interactions between physicians and patients in the hospital without physical contact, thus decreasing risks of infection for vulnerable populations.[14] Certified bodies and frequent auditing are needed to incorporate appropriate trainings for such telehealth programs to ensure safety and efficacy.[15]

Virtual reality (VR) facilitates the user's perception of reality by creating a computer-generated environment using head-mounted displays, wall projectors, and touch-sensitive motors. VR has been explored for the treatment of a range of medical conditions, including anxiety, phobias, obesity, chronic pain, and eating disorders because of its capacity "to modulate subjective experience, offer respite from the confining nature of medical wards, or augment or replace analgesics in pain management."[16] In a randomized controlled trial that recruited 90 women with binge eating disorder at a rehab center, 44.4% of patients who used virtual reality were able to improve or maintain weight loss compared with 10.4% of patients in control conditions.[16] In the management of mental illness, VR-based cognitive and vocational training has been shown to improve cognitive outcomes.[17]

Moreover, simulated patients have been used in medical training.[15] Augmented reality (AR) refers to the enhancement of real-world experiences via the addition of computer-generated sensory information[18] and has been considered for real-time interactions with anatomy in surgical training and for consultations or mentoring with specialists independent of location.[18]

Remote Patient Monitoring and Remote Physiologic Monitoring

RPM uses mobile applications and sensory devices to collect community health care data or deliver real-time patient information to practitioners.[5] Expectations associated with remote patient monitoring include decreased hospital use, improved patient compliance, improved satisfaction with health services, and improved quality of life.

In addition to its usage in urgent services and ICUs for monitoring vitals,[5] RPM allows chronic diseases to be increasingly managed at home versus at a long-term-care facility. Physicians are able to monitor vitals and other patient data to prevent emergency room visits.[10] Improvements in chronic disease management are especially significant in the United States, where "more than 70% of deaths are associated with chronic diseases and approximately 75% of annual health care expenses are used on persons with chronic conditions."[19] Based on findings from 58 systematic reviews, RPM has been shown to improve mortality and quality of life, and reduce hospital admissions.[20] A meta-analysis of 11 randomized controlled trials showed that telehealth exercise-based cardiac rehabilitation is at least comparable with center-based rehabilitation for reducing cardiovascular risk factors and improving functional capacity.[21]

RPM also improves health care engagement of patients and family members and shows promise in encouraging patients to achieve and maintain health goals.[19] It is specifically helpful for monitoring pediatric patients with type 1 diabetes via alerts during hypoglycemic or hyperglycemic incidences. For cardiac patients, cardiovascular implantable devices have been shown to decrease incidences of adverse cardiac events.[14] Findings based on 53 systematic reviews showed that telehealth-mediated self-management support for long-term conditions such as diabetes, heart failure, asthma, chronic obstructive pulmonary disease, and cancer is not consistently better than in-person support, although no reviews showed evidence of harm. Reviews more consistently showed reductions in mortality and hospital admissions for patients with heart failure and improvements in glycemic control for type 2 diabetics.[22] Furthermore, a meta-analysis comprising 25 studies showed evidence that telehealth-mediated dietary interventions for adults with chronic conditions improved diet quality, fruit and vegetable intake, and sodium intake.[23]

Starting from January 1, 2020, hospitals and health systems receive more Medicare reimbursements for RPM services. In its final rule on chronic care remote physiologic monitoring,[24] the Centers for Medicare & Medicaid Services (CMS) has allowed RPM to be furnished as a service "incident to" under general supervision, defined by CMS as service performed under the supervision of a qualified health care professional and billed to Medicare in the name of that professional. As such, CMS allows Current Procedural Terminology code 99457 to be billed for the first 20 minutes per month of RPM services and also added a new code 99458 for patients receiving an additional 20 minutes of mHealth services in a given month.

Overall

The cost, patient adherence, technology use, and effectiveness of telehealth vary depending on the technology and specialty.[14] Based on 58 systematic reviews that evaluated the impact of telehealth based on clinical outcomes, use, or cost, telehealth is most consistently beneficial when used for communication, counseling, or RPM of chronic diseases.[20] For example, a systematic review of 22 studies showed that telehealth interventions for cancer survivors minimizes disruptions to patients' lives and facilitates personalized care.[25] Uses of pediatric telehealth include acute-care visits, pretransport assessment and stabilization of those in critical condition, RPM, and specialty consultations.[26]

Cost of telehealth

Costs associated with the setup and maintenance of telehealth systems should also be considered, including use of telehealth personnel, costs of consultations, information technology support, equipment licenses, connectivity charges, and medical records management.[7]

An analysis of episode-level costs based on a cross-sectional retrospective study that included visits for the most common telehealth diagnoses (sinusitis, upper respiratory infections, urinary tract infections, conjunctivitis, bronchitis, pharyngitis, influenza, cough, dermatitis, nausea/vomiting/diarrhea, and ear pain) showed similar follow-up rates (with follow-up rate being a possible indication for misdiagnoses or treatment failure) between patients evaluated virtually and those evaluated traditionally; lower treatment cost per episode of care (defined as the initial visit plus the following 3 weeks) for virtual visits, which also depended on the condition; lower laboratory testing rates after virtual visits; and higher antibiotic prescription rates after virtual visits.[8]

Using claims and enrollment data from approximately 300,000 patients, net annual spending on acute respiratory illness increased $45 per telehealth user. Only an estimate of 12% of telehealth visits replaced visits to other providers, whereas 88% represented new use.[27]

Why telehealth works

Improved outcomes, preference, ease of use, cost savings, improved communication, travel time, and improved self-management were the most prevalent factors for choosing telehealth.[28] Specifically, time savings and increased accessibility were noted reasons for scheduled virtual visits.[11] The usage of mobile health and the market for mobile applications are increasing because of the convenience of size and mobility.[5,7] There is widespread interest in using phone and Internet-based telehealth among patients with chronic diseases.[29] With improvements in mortality for premature infants, patients with cancer, and patients with cardiovascular diseases, there is an increasing demand for health services. Management via telehealth encourages patients to participate in their own care and allows physicians to intervene as needed.[14,19,25]

Social adaptability, including patient and staff acceptance, will facilitate telehealth adoption. Patient acceptance and confidence in telehealth are highest for emergencies and higher for treatment than for diagnosis. Rural participants responded most positively and the scores within families tend to be similar.[7] The acceptance of telehealth for patients with chronic diseases increases with younger age, higher levels of education, familiarity, perceived usefulness, perceived ease of use, and satisfaction.[17] Among survey participants from telehealth users of scheduled video visits, 91.3% reported satisfaction. Among the dissatisfied, most cited technical issues. Ease of use was agreed on by 86.7%, 91.0% reported having had enough time with the provider, 82.7% perceived the same level of care as in in-person visits, and 87.6% perceived at least an hour of time saved.[11] Qualitative interviews conducted with patients who declined to participate in another telehealth study showed that major concerns include threats to identity, independence, and self-care; requirements of technical proficiency and the ability to operate equipment; and experiences of service disruptions.[17]

Equally important is staff acceptance, which is influenced by the staff's working environment, the manner of introduction, personal experiences, training, support, and the process of integration for routine care.[30,31] A common concern is the belief that the use of virtual visits will decrease patient-provider relationships.[7] Initial impressions of telehealth are an important factor. One study showed that nurses tended to be uncertain about the role of telehealth, which was intensified by the limitations and apparent contradictions of current research about its cost and clinical effectiveness. The adaptability of nurses was also affected by training on identifying suitable patients, effective monitoring and triage, duration of use, and the expected benefits and drawbacks.[30] A survey on implementation of robotic telepresence showed that NICU nurses thought that physicians were easily accessible via robotic telepresence, adequately involved, and supportive of both nurses and patients.[14]

Current problems

The success and availability of telehealth depends on the speed of data transmission, reliability, and security.[7] AR and VR are currently limited by computer power, battery life, the size of devices, and portability.[18] In order to successfully engage patients and improve communication, technologies must accommodate to the user's needs. Besides the patient's condition, the chosen platform should be based on the patient's age, education, interests, physical capabilities, familiarity, access to technology, the amount of support for self-care, and functional independence.[19]

Policy and regulations are often disjointed at the federal and state levels. In the United States, because states currently define their own policies, there is a wide range of telehealth definitions and reimbursement policies. Similarly, health care systems vary from country to country.[19] Although there is ongoing effort to increase telehealth use and reimbursement, health care providers continue to encounter conflicting or vague policies for the requirements for insurance claims, practice standards, and licensure,[10,26] and there is no consistent pattern of coverage and reimbursement for the variety of applications.[7,12,26] Lack of cost-benefit analysis also hinders the development of telehealth policies federally as well as the adoption and growth of telehealth programs.[19]

In terms of cost, further research is needed to confirm that higher follow-up visit rates do not occur as a result of unresolved symptoms or because telehealth is used before in-person visits.[8] In addition, within the United States, many payers do not yet "recognize the home as a reimbursable site of care."[19]

Considering the expansion of pediatric telehealth, a survey administered by the Supporting Pediatrics Research on Outcomes and Utilization of Telehealth program with 56 responses from mostly academic medical centers using pediatric telehealth identified barriers including licensing requirements, provider interest, and limitations of training resources.[26]

There is also a lack of quality monitoring for telehealth practices. There are concerns of whether physicians can provide accurate diagnoses without a physical in-person examination, whether patients receive appropriate laboratory testing after the visit, and whether antibiotics are overprescribed.[8] If data from RPM and other telehealth technologies are used to make clinical decisions, the physicians must be able to rely on the precision and accuracy of gathered data.[19] Most successful telehealth models require an extensive team to coordinate care to translate processed data from various devices into clinical action.[19]

Privacy and security concerns are also a major consideration in the deployment of telehealth. Privacy risks involve a lack of control on the collection, use, and disclosure of sensitive personal information.[32] Routine transmissions from a medical device may be collected and stored by the device or the app developer in addition to the health care provider. Security concerns depend on the platform. A patient participating in a video consultation may be concerned about the presence of others in the room, whereas someone using RPM technology may have concerns about the reliability of the device.[7] Specifically, in telehealth models where 1 end of the communication is the patient, no Health Insurance Portability and Accountability Act regulation or required safeguards are in place, magnifying existing concerns.[32] Patients may perceive security features as nuisances if they do not perceive some of their protected health information (PHI) to be sensitive.[33] At present, federal and state guidelines for telehealth security and privacy are not standardized, leaving considerable gaps.[34]

In addition, there are limitations of current literature. Past studies tend to consist of people who were already positively disposed to telehealth.[19] An analysis of 110 telehealth studies on chronic diseases, with 108 reporting positive outcomes, showed that the studies averaged a length of 6 months and there were few studies of cost-effectiveness.[19] Published literature is lacking, particularly in pediatrics, with previous studies largely focused on acceptability or patient characteristics rather than outcomes.[8] Other areas that require more extensive research include the management of serious pediatric conditions, triage in urgent or primary care, and teledermatology outcomes.

SUMMARY

Telehealth shows enormous potential as a new way for clinicians to reach patients remotely, often in the comfort of their homes. However, wider adoption of telehealth would require careful consideration of patient preferences, safety, effectiveness, medicolegal, and operational issues.

DISCLOSURE

The authors have nothing to disclose.

REFERENCES

1. Health Resources & Services Administration. Telehealth Programs. Available at: https://www.hrsa.gov/rural-health/telehealth/index.html. Accessed September 17, 2019.
2. WHO. Monitoring and Evaluating Digital Health Interventions: A Practical Guide to Conducting Research and Assessment.; 2016. doi:CC BY-NC-SA 3.0 IGO.
3. Kvedar J, Coye MJ, Everett W. Connected health: A review of technologies and strategies to improve patient care with telemedicine and telehealth. Health Aff 2014;33(2):194–9.
4. Caulfield BM, Donnelly SC. What is connected health and why will it change your practice? QJM 2013;106(8):703–7.
5. Weinstein RS, Lopez AM, Joseph BA, et al. Telemedicine, telehealth, and mobile health applications that work: Opportunities and barriers. Am J Med 2014;127(3): 183–7.
6. Eysenbach G. What is e-health? J Med Internet Res 2001;3(2):e20.
7. Sikka N, Paradise S, Shu M. Telehealth in emergency medicine: a primer. 2014.
8. Gordon AS, Adamson WC, DeVries AR. Virtual visits for acute, nonurgent care: A claims analysis of episode-level utilization. J Med Internet Res 2017;19(2):1–11.
9. Marcin JP, Shaikh U, Steinhorn RH. Addressing health disparities in rural communities using telehealth. Pediatr Res 2016;79(1–2):169–76.
10. Marcoux RM, Vogenberg FR. Telehealth: applications from a legal and regulatory perspective. P T. 2016;41(9):567–70.

11. Powell RE, Stone D, Hollander JE. Patient and health system experience with implementation of an enterprise-wide telehealth scheduled video visit program: Mixed-methods study. J Med Internet Res 2018;20(2):1–7.

12. Brophy PD. Overview on the challenges and benefits of using telehealth tools in a pediatric population. Adv Chronic Kidney Dis 2017;24(1):17–21.

13. van Galen LS, Wang CJ, Nanayakkara PWB, et al. Telehealth requires expansion of physicians' communication competencies training. Med Teach 2019;41(6): 714–5.

14. Banbury A, Nancarrow S, Dart J, et al. Telehealth interventions delivering home-based support group videoconferencing: Systematic review. J Med Internet Res 2018;20(2). https://doi.org/10.2196/jmir.8090.

15. Sasangohar F, Davis E, Kash BA, et al. Remote patient monitoring and telemedicine in neonatal and pediatric settings: Scoping literature review. J Med Internet Res 2018;20(12):1–9.

16. Dascal J, Reid M, Ishak WW, et al. Virtual reality and medical inpatients: a systematic review of randomized, Controlled Trials. Innov Clin Neurosci 2017;14(1): 14–21.

17. Lawes-Wickwar S, McBain H, Mulligan K. Application and effectiveness of telehealth to support severe mental illness management: systematic review. JMIR Ment Health 2018;5(4):e62.

18. Khor WS, Baker B, Amin K, et al. Augmented and virtual reality in surgery—the digital surgical environment: applications, limitations and legal pitfalls. Ann Transl Med 2016;4(23):454.

19. Dinesen B, Nonnecke B, Lindeman D, et al. Personalized telehealth in the future: A global research agenda. J Med Internet Res 2016;18(3). https://doi.org/10.2196/jmir.5257.

20. Totten AM, Womack DM, Eden KB, et al. Telehealth: mapping the evidence for patient outcomes from systematic reviews [Internet]. Rockville (MD): Agency for Healthcare Research and Quality (US); 2016. Available at: https://www.ncbi.nlm.nih.gov/books/NBK379320/.

21. Rawstorn JC, Gant N, Direito A, et al. Telehealth exercise-based cardiac rehabilitation: A systematic review and meta-analysis. Heart 2016;102(15):1183–92.

22. Hanlon P, Daines L, Campbell C, et al. Telehealth interventions to support self-management of long-term conditions: A systematic metareview of diabetes, heart failure, asthma, chronic obstructive pulmonary disease, and cancer. J Med Internet Res 2017;19(5). https://doi.org/10.2196/jmir.6688.

23. Kelly JT, Reidlinger DP, Hoffmann TC, et al. Telehealth methods to deliver dietary interventions in adults with chronic disease: A systematic review and meta-analysis1,2. Am J Clin Nutr 2016;104(6):1693–702.

24. Centers for Medicare & Medicaid Services. Document 2019-24086. Office of the federal register 2019. Available at: https://www.federalregister.gov/documents/2019/11/15/2019-24086/medicare-program-cy-2020-revisions-to-payment-policies-under-the-physician-fee-schedule-and-other. Accessed February 10, 2020.

25. Cox A, Lucas G, Marcu A, et al. Cancer survivors' experience with telehealth: A systematic review and thematic synthesis. J Med Internet Res 2017;19(1):1–19.

26. Olson CA, Mcswain SD, Curfman AL, et al. The current pediatric telehealth landscape. Pediatrics 2018;141(3). https://doi.org/10.1542/peds.2017-2334.

27. Ashwood JS, Mehrotra A, Cowling D, et al. Direct-to-consumer telehealth may increase access to care but does not decrease spending. Health Aff 2017;36(3): 485–91.

28. Kruse CS, Krowski N, Rodriguez B, et al. Telehealth and patient satisfaction: a systematic review and narrative analysis. BMJ Open 2017;1–12. https://doi.org/10.1136/bmjopen-2017-016242.

29. Edwards L, Thomas C, Gregory A, et al. Are people with chronic diseases interested in using telehealth? A cross-sectional postal survey. J Med Internet Res 2014;16(5):1–16.

30. Taylor J, Coates E, Brewster L, et al. Examining the use of telehealth in community nursing: Identifying the factors affecting frontline staff acceptance and telehealth adoption. J Adv Nurs 2015;71(2):326–37.

31. Koivunen M, Saranto K. Nursing professionals' experiences of the facilitators and barriers to the use of telehealth applications: a systematic review of qualitative studies. Scand J Caring Sci 2018;32(1):24–44.

32. Hall BJL, Mcgraw D. For telehealth to succeed, privacy and security risks must be identified and addressed. Health Aff (Millwood) 2014;33(2):216–21.

33. Wang CJ, Huang DJ. The HIPAA conundrum in the era of mobile health and communications. JAMA 2013;310(11):1121–2.

34. Tuckson RV, Edmunds M, Hodgkins ML. Telehealth. N Engl J Med 2017;377:1585–93.

The Role of Text Messaging and Telehealth Messaging Apps

Sashikumar Ganapathy, MB BCh Bao, MRCPCH(UK), MSc[a,b],
Dirk F. de Korne, PhD, MSc[b,c,d,e],
Ng Kee Chong, MBBS, MMed(Paeds), FRCPCH, AMS(Singapore)[a,b],
Josip Car, MD, PhD[f,*]

KEYWORDS

• Text-based messaging • Applications • Telehealth • Legal issues • Technology

KEY POINTS

• The rapid advancement of technology experienced worldwide in the recent past continues to leave a significant effect wherever the technology is applied.

• Currently, various telecommunication tools, such as the Internet, email, and videoconferencing, are used in the health care context to exchange information among doctors and patients regarding different health problems, ranging from acute to chronic conditions, such as minor injuries, febrile conditions, weight management, smoking cessation, medication adherence, depression, anxiety, and stress.

• One particular telecommunication tool that is gaining wider popularity is the use of text messaging, whose use comes with low costs, quick delivery, increased safety, and lower intrusiveness compared with telephone calls.

INTRODUCTION

The rapid advancement of technology experienced worldwide in the recent past continues to leave a significant effect wherever the technology is applied. Currently, various telecommunication tools, such as the Internet, email, and videoconferencing, are used in the health care context to exchange information among doctors and

[a] KK Women's & Children's Hospital, 100, Bukit Timah Road 229899 Singapore; [b] Duke-NUS School of Medicine, Singapore, Singapore; [c] Medical Innovation & Care Transformation, KK Women's & Children's Hospital, Singapore, Singapore; [d] Erasmus School of Health Policy and Management, Erasmus University Rotterdam, Rotterdam, Netherlands; [e] Care & Welfare, SVRZ Cares in Zeeland, Middelburg, SVRZ, Koudekerkseweg 143, Middelburg 4335 SM, Netherlands; [f] Centre for Population Health Sciences, Lee Kong Chian School of Medicine, Nanyang Technological University, Singapore, Clinical Sciences Building, 11 Mandalay Road, Singapore 308232, Singapore
* Corresponding author.
E-mail address: josip.car@ntu.edu.sg
Twitter: @dirkdekorne (D.F.K.); @ejosipcar (J.C.)

Pediatr Clin N Am 67 (2020) 613–621
https://doi.org/10.1016/j.pcl.2020.04.002
0031-3955/20/© 2020 Elsevier Inc. All rights reserved.

patients regarding different health problems, ranging from acute to chronic conditions, such as minor injuries, febrile conditions, weight management, smoking cessation, medication adherence, depression, anxiety, and stress.[1] Indeed, "(t)he rapid expansion of mobile health (mHealth) programs through text messaging provides an opportunity to improve health knowledge, behaviors, and clinical outcomes, particularly among hard-to-reach populations."[2] Rathbone and Prescott[3] state that "Studies have found that 31% of mobile phone owners use them to access health information; 19% have also installed a mobile app that relates to a current medical condition or to manage their health and well-being." Another study showed that "over 56% of health-care settings use mHealth to aid clinical practice."[4] One particular telecommunication tool that is, gaining wider popularity is the use of text messaging, whose use comes with low costs, quick delivery, increased safety, and lower intrusiveness compared with telephone calls.[5]

TEXT MESSAGING IN TELEHEALTH

Currently, text messaging is being used in telemedicine and telehealth where patients and doctors use their different electronic gadgets, such as personal computers, tablets, or mobile phones, to communicate through text-based messaging transmitted as short message services (SMS) over networks of mobile operators or the Internet. This is where mobile and computer applications, such as WhatsApp, WeChat, FaceTime, Messenger, Line, and Viber, among others, come into use. This article examines the role of these and other text messaging apps in telehealth, with an overview on whether these apps meet HIPAA and other considerations.

As is the case with any other set-up, people will use the most efficient, convenient, and cost-effective platform available. The use of text messaging services and apps comes in with what most of their users desire, particularly concerning the cost in terms of money and time, and convenience, the latter arising from the ability of mobile devices to have several communications tools/apps in a single mobile device.[1] Because of their low cost and reliance, text messaging apps are widely used to share information used for various purposes, including administrative, health disease management, education, telepathology, health and behavior change, diagnoses and management, triage, home monitoring, or screening.[6] According to Kamel and colleagues,[7] telemedicine services implemented in urology, where patients perform video visits, have saved patients of Los Angeles VA Hospital considerable costs in the money and time they spent per visit. Used this way, WhatsApp, for instance, has been able to eliminate geographic constraints that are common concerning physical visits to health service providers. The use of WhatsApp and generally other telehealth apps encourage not only seeking initial clinical but also ongoing expert clinical care among health care professionals.[8] Hence, one of the roles of text messaging and messaging apps in telehealth is reducing the cost while improving the convenience of sharing information.

Text messaging and messaging apps also play a key role in strengthening health care systems. Besides enhancing the accessibility of health care services, text messaging and messaging apps can open up access to health care services for patients in remote areas. As health care services get closer to the people, more patients are likely to benefit from emergency referrals, whereas other groups of people, such as community workers, midwives, especially those in remote areas, are able to receive the support that is otherwise limited or absent.[2,9] The use of text messaging and messaging apps also makes it easier for community health workers to collect data remotely.[2]

The host of services and capacities of mobile devices will also benefit users in various ways, such as to support various health interventions, among them health promotion and disease prevention, treatment compliance, health information systems and point-of-care support, data collection and disease surveillance, and emergency medical response.[2] For instance, the messaging services and apps enhance the delivery of information related to health practices and prevention of diseases, thereby promoting healthy behaviors. Besides, patients and providers benefit from common uses of text messaging services and apps, including setting and/or passing reminders for appointments, monitoring dermatologic lesions, remote screening and diagnosis, creation of patient self-reports, storages and forwarding of results, skin self-examination and burns, health behavior reminders concerning the use sunscreen, and monitoring compliance for prevention and treatment.[2,3,6,10] Health professionals, such as doctors and community health workers, also benefit from clinical support that telemedicine is able to offer concerning functions, such as access to real-time data, and creating clinic and hospital records on the outbreak of diseases through monitoring of patient attendances. Concerning this role, some of the text-messaging initiatives that are in use include Text4baby, TXT4Tots, SmokeFreeTXT, QuitNowTXT, Health Alerts On-the-Go, Text Alert Toolkit, and SmokeFree Moms.[2]

Evidence exists on the acceptance, usage, and effectiveness of text messaging programs in telehealth. Studies on the use of SMS reminders show that the use of text messaging help improves patient-medical compliance, and that text messages make a better choice for users based on ease of use, low costs of use, and rapid and automated delivery of messages.[11] According to research by the US Department of Health and Human Services, descriptive studies have provided insights into not only patient preferences for text messaging concerning the receipt of health information and reminders but also retention in health interventions after enrollment,[2] hence the reason text messaging can safely be made a regular practice.

APPLICATIONS IN ADULT CARE

For telehealth in the general (adult) population, messaging apps have been used to stimulate compliance and self-management in patients with chronic issues. Automatic text reminders for ambulatory visits are common, but also reminders for tests and vaccinations.[12,13] Maugalian and colleagues[14] reviewed the use of text messaging in oncology, and described examples of successful text messaging interventions, including addressing behavioral change, attendance to screening and follow-up appointments, adherence to treatment, and assessment of symptoms and quality of life.

Huo and colleagues[15] show how a text message intervention resulted in better glycemic control in patients with diabetes mellitus and coronary heart disease. Having the text messages sent by the patient's family or friends showed an increased effect on health-related lifestyle issues[16,17] and mental health.[18–20] Comparable examples are known from smoking cessation,[21,22] addiction,[23,24] and patients on hemodialysis.[25]

SEXINFO, an innovation developed by the US Agency for Healthcare Research and Quality Health Care Innovations Exchange with the intention of creating awareness about the high rates of spread of gonorrhea in San Francisco, proved effective in the use, sharing, and satisfaction with messages, and a high number of inquiries and referrals.[26] One great aspect of the SEXINFO innovation is that it capitalized on the inseparability concerning access and use of mobile technology to reach the target audience. In Australia, the use of text message interventions to teach youths about sexually transmitted infections showed greater use compared with emails; "the use of text messages related to sexual health suggests that text messaging offers promise for reaching teens about health information, referrals, and testing reminders."[2]

In New York, text messaging interventions used for delivery of immunization reminders among English- and Spanish-speaking expectant women and parents of adolescents showed an improved rate of vaccinations and that the parents of adolescents were uniformly satisfied based on simplicity, brevity, and personalization.[27,28] The same positive result of the interventions showed that pregnant women were interested in the programs concerning encouragement to take vaccines and talk to clinicians during pregnancy.[27] The same can apply for other categories of people given the ever-increasing use of mobile technology across the globe, including patients with human immunodeficiency virus/AIDS for whom evidence shows that reminders are helpful in adherence to medications and hence suppression of viral load.[29]

APPLICATIONS IN PEDIATRIC CARE

As in health care in general, the use of text messaging has also been applied in pediatric care only recently. One of the first studies on text messaging was done in Denmark and indicated that SMS reminders reduced nonattendance at the pediatric outpatient clinic.[30]

In 2012, a systematic review studied the evidence using text messaging as a tool to deliver healthy lifestyle behavior intervention programs in pediatric and adolescent populations.[31] They found 37 relevant articles and concluded the high potential of text messaging–delivered health care behavior interventions that work as a reminder system for chronic disease management in these populations.

In 2013, a Harvard qualitative study using focus groups concluded that "text messaging is a promising medium for supporting and encouraging pediatric obesity-related behavior changes."[32] Similarly, a Johns Hopkins survey indicated that "caregivers of children would be interested in communicating with healthcare providers following an ED visit."[33] In a trauma resilience and recovery program, mental health symptoms postinjury were tracked via a 30-day text messaging program and screening for post-traumatic stress disorder via a questionnaire was completed via telephone screens.[34] Standardized text messages improved the 30-day follow-up for American College of Surgeons National Surgical Quality Improvement Program scores.[35] In pediatric tonsillectomy patients, text messaging was used to improve communication and overall experience.[36] In pediatric asthma, real-time capture of peak flow rate meter readings was done with SMS.[37]

In diabetes care, Stephens and colleagues[38] show how behavioral intervention technologies and artificial intelligence could help in pediatric obesity and prediabetes treatment support. Moreover, encouragement for influenza vaccines was successfully given by text messaging in a pediatric population.[39–41]

The role of text messaging for disease monitoring was also studied in childhood nephrotic syndrome.[42] Text messages soliciting home urine protein results, symptoms, and medication adherence were sent to a caregiver who responded by texting. The system reliably captured number of disease relapses and time-to-remission compared with data collected by conventional visits.

Text messaging may also play an important role in obtaining and using patient-reported outcomes. Mellor and colleagues[43] show that text messaging permits valid assessment of the Pediatric International Knee Documentation Committee and Pediatric Functional Activity Brief Scale scores in adolescents.[43] They conclude that "questionnaire delivery by automated text messaging allows asynchronous response and may increase compliance and reduce the labor cost of collecting PRO's [patient-reported outcomes]."

In a study in patients after neonatal intensive care unit discharge, Flores-Fenlon and colleagues[44] concluded that smartphones and text messaging were associated with higher parent quality-of-life scores and enrollment in early intervention.[44]

USE OF CROSS-PLATFORM MESSAGING APPLICATIONS

Such apps as WhatsApp, WeChat, and Line are ubiquitous cross-platform messaging and voice-over Internet protocol/Internet protocol freeware services.

Currently, WhatsApp Messenger is one of the most widely used mobile apps in telehealth; however, various sources have indicated that this application and likes have serious limitations with regard to privacy and data security. Many attribute the widespread use of WhatsApp Messenger to its extensive capabilities, such as to share high-quality photographs, videos, and voice messages, and to make voice and video calls, videos on top of text-based messages. In addition, WhatsApp Messenger uses an Internet connection that can use a mobile data plan or Wi-Fi, which makes it more affordable than the conventional SMS modality. With quality, reliability, and low cost, WhatsApp Messenger has become one of the most preferred messaging apps among patients and health professionals because the information shared (images and videos) is of sufficient detail as would be needed to make adequate diagnosis and initial treatment, leading to better efficacy compared with other modalities that can serve the same purpose.[6] The WhatsApp Group feature that is part of WhatsApp Messenger is also an excellent platform for text blasting/bulk messaging because it allows sharing information to 256 people at once, or by the use of the app's Broadcast Lists where information can be repeatedly shared to preselected and saved list of recipients, eliminating the need to select the recipients each time.[7] In this case, for instance, a health professional can create a group and add relevant members, after which the professional will instantly share a piece of educational or related information to all members, which is faster than having to share the information to each recipient individually.

Results of research examining the usefulness of WhatsApp in clinical decision-making and patient care showed that the mobile app is a "low-cost and fast technology with the potential of facilitating clinical communications, enhancing learning, and improving patient care while preserving their privacy."[7] When used on patients battling with smoking relapse, WhatsApp provides enhanced discussion and social support, which proved effective in helping the patients reduce relapse to rates of 2 and 6 months as the authors continue to narrate. Additionally, when used among emergency surgery teams in a London hospital, WhatsApp was attributed to a flattened hierarchy that allowed all participants (students, residents, and experienced consultants) to actively and freely contribute to the discussions. These authors also found WhatsApp to be a better platform for case discourses, increasing awareness on patient-related information, improving the efficiency of the handover process, and reducing the duration of ancient morning handover processes among orthopedic residents. These are just a few examples of the situations where the use of WhatsApp in health care has proved beneficial. Various bodies, however, suggest taking serious steps to ensure compliance with data protection laws when introducing text messaging services. To safeguard data privacy and confidentiality, mobile messaging should only take place through a secure health care messaging application, and in Europe the National Health Service has provided detailed instructions for its practice.

In Asia WeChat and Line are the WhatsApp equivalent. In China, WeChat is used to expand human immunodeficiency virus testing by reaching key parts of the population, among them nonheterosexuals who rarely do testing.[45] However, there are considerable security concerns. The population whom the said study targeted were apprehensive about using the platform and participating in the intervention for fear that the information shared through the app would reach their families, which would then have exposed their sexual orientation.

LEGAL IMPLICATIONS

Despite the increasing use and promising potential benefits, the use of text messaging and messaging apps in telemedicine is limited by whether they are compliant with US HIPAA regulations, Europe's General Data Protection Regulation, and Singapore's Personal Data Protection Act, among other bodies. For instance, HIPAA is particular about sharing of protected health information as a text message.[7] HIPAA's security rule includes specific security standards for the disclosure and storage of electronic health information and requires safeguarding of PHI [protected health information]. This means that before a messaging app is used, its security standards must meet some threshold. Besides, texting is shown to have a unique set of risks that without management compromise the privacy and security of the shared information. For example, this could happen if the mobile devices are lost or recycled.[46]

In a study reported in 2014, pediatric hospitalists were surveyed on their use of text messaging. Forty-six percent of the 97 respondents worried privacy laws can be violated by sending/receiving text messages, and 30% reported having protected health information in text messages.[47] However, only 11% reported their institution offered encryption software for text messaging.

In pediatric dermatology, text messaging and cell phone cameras have facilitated curbside consultations and a recent survey indicated that they increase access and promote collegiality; but they are also usually not compensated, consume considerable time, risk liability exposure for providers, and potentially compromise confidentiality.[48]

The information a patient discloses to a physician is confidential and should be treated as such.[40] Hence, before any of these apps are put into wide telemedical use, a thorough evaluation is needed to ensure consistency and compliance with ethical practices. Notably, HIPAA does not bar the use of any mode of communication, including texting, but care should be taken to enhance the safety and privacy of information shared.[8,46] Such apps as WhatsApp Messenger are deploying end-to-end encryption that enhances the safety of information shared, which can make them among the HIPAA-compliant messaging apps. Generally, HIPAA recommends using messaging apps under secure encrypted networks with access and audit controls.[49]

This paper has discussed the role of text messaging and messaging applications including technical and legal issues. The reviews of current examples of text messaging in adult and pediatric practice show uptake has been increasing substantially in the past 3 years, especially to stimulate adherence and self-management in patients with chronic diseases. In pediatric care text messaging has been used for behavior intervention and outcomes tracking. Although applications are promising, especially efficiencies and selected, the potential of nonsynchronic messaging in the formal delivery of care is still in the neonatal phase compared with its grown-up existence in day-to-day modern life.

REFERENCES

1. Shah O, Matlaga B. Emerging technologies in renal stone management, an issue of urologic clinics, EBook. Elsevier Health Sciences; 2019.

2. US Department of Health and Human Services. Health resources and services administration. Using health text messages to improve consumer health knowledge, behaviors, and outcomes: an environmental scan. Rockville (MD): US Department of Health and Human Services; 2014.
3. Rathbone AL, Prescott J. The use of mobile apps and SMS messaging as physical and mental health interventions: systematic review. J Med Internet Res 2017; 19(8):e295.
4. Franko OI, Tirrell TF. Smartphone app use among medical providers in ACGME training programs. J Med Syst 2012;36(5):3135–9.
5. Kannisto KA, Koivunen MH, Välimäki MA. Use of mobile phone text message reminders in health care services: a narrative literature review. J Med Internet Res 2014;16(10):e222.
6. Morris C, Scott RE, Mars M. Instant messaging in dermatology: a literature review. Stud Health Technol Inform 2018;254:70–6.
7. Kamel Boulos M, Giustini D, Wheeler S. Instagram and WhatsApp in health and healthcare: an overview. Future Internet 2016;8(3):37.
8. Mars M, Scott RE. WhatsApp in clinical practice: a literature. The promise of new technologies in an age of new health challenges. Stud Health Technol Inform 2016;231:82–90.
9. Giordano V, Koch H, Godoy-Santos A, et al. WhatsApp messenger as an adjunctive tool for telemedicine: an overview. Interact J Med Res 2017;6(2):e11.
10. Schilling L, Bennett G, Bull S, et al. Text messaging in healthcare research toolkit. Center for Research in Implementation Science and Prevention (CRISP), University of Colorado School of Medicine; 2013.
11. Schwebel FJ, Larimer ME. Using text message reminders in health care services: a narrative literature review. Internet Interv 2018;13:82–104.
12. Esteban-Vasallo M, Domínguez-Berjón M, García-Riolobos C, et al. Effect of mobile phone text messaging for improving the uptake of influenza vaccination in patients with rare diseases. Vaccine 2019;37(36):5257–64.
13. Lee HY, Lee MH, Sharratt M, et al. Development of a mobile health intervention to promote Papanicolaou tests and human papillomavirus vaccination in an underserved immigrant population: a culturally targeted and individually tailored text messaging approach. JMIR Mhealth Uhealth 2019;7(6):e13256.
14. Mougalian SS, Gross CP, Hall EK. Text messaging in oncology: A review of the landscape. JCO clinical cancer informatics 2018;2:1–9.
15. Huo X, Spatz ES, Ding Q, et al. Design and rationale of the Cardiovascular Health and Text Messaging (CHAT) Study and the CHAT-Diabetes Mellitus (CHAT-DM) Study: two randomised controlled trials of text messaging to improve secondary prevention for coronary heart disease and diabetes. BMJ 2017;7(12):e018302.
16. Haider R, Hyun K, Cheung NW, et al. Effect of lifestyle focused text messaging on risk factor modification in patients with diabetes and coronary heart disease: a sub-analysis of the TEXT ME study. Diabetes Res Clin Pract 2019;153:184–90.
17. Mayberry LS, Bergner EM, Harper KJ, et al. Text messaging to engage friends/family in diabetes self-management support: acceptability and potential to address disparities. J Am Med Inform Assoc 2019;26(10):1099–108.
18. Stevens GJ, Hammond TE, Brownhill S, et al. SMS SOS: a randomized controlled trial to reduce self-harm and suicide attempts using SMS text messaging. BMC Psychiatry 2019;19(1):117.
19. Thomas K, Bendtsen M. Mental health promotion among university students using text messaging: protocol for a randomized controlled trial of a mobile phone–based intervention. JMIR Res Protoc 2019;8(8):e12396.

20. Xu DR, Xiao S, He H, et al. Lay health supporters aided by mobile text messaging to improve adherence, symptoms, and functioning among people with schizophrenia in a resource-poor community in rural China (LEAN): A randomized controlled trial. PLoS Med 2019;16(4):e1002785.

21. Cartujano-Barrera F, Arana-Chicas E, Ramírez-Mantilla M, et al. "Every day I think about your messages": assessing text messaging engagement among Latino smokers in a mobile cessation program. Patient Prefer Adherence 2019;13:1213.

22. Nolan MB, Warner MA, Jacobs MA, et al. Feasibility of a perioperative text messaging smoking cessation program for surgical patients. Anesth Analg 2019;129(3):e73–6.

23. Bendtsen M. Text messaging interventions for reducing alcohol consumption among harmful and hazardous drinkers: protocol for a systematic review and meta-analysis. JMIR Res Protoc 2019;8(4):e12898.

24. Mastroleo NR, Celio MA, Barnett NP, et al. Feasibility and acceptability of a motivational intervention combined with text messaging for alcohol and sex risk reduction with emergency department patients: a pilot trial. Addict Res Theory 2019;27(2):85–94.

25. Stevenson J, Campbell KL, Brown M, et al. Targeted, structured text messaging to improve dietary and lifestyle behaviours for people on maintenance haemodialysis (KIDNEYTEXT): study protocol for a randomised controlled trial. BMJ Open 2019;9(5):e023545.

26. Levine D, McCright J, Dobkin L, et al. SEXINFO: a sexual health text messaging service for San Francisco youth. Am J Public Health 2008;98(3):393–5.

27. Kharbanda EO, Vargas CY, Castaño PM, et al. Exploring pregnant women's views on influenza vaccination and educational text messages. Prev Med 2011;52(1):75–7.

28. Stockwell MS, Kharbanda EO, Martinez RA, et al. Text4Health: impact of text message reminder–recalls for pediatric and adolescent immunizations. Am J Public Health 2012;102(2):e15–21.

29. Lauffenburger JC, Choudhry NK. Text messaging and patient engagement in an increasingly mobile world. Circulation 2016;133(6):555–6.

30. Kruse L, Hansen L, Olesen C. Non-attendance at a pediatric outpatient clinic. SMS text messaging improves attendance. Ugeskr Laeger 2009;171(17):1372–5.

31. Militello LK, Kelly SA, Melnyk BM. Systematic review of text-messaging interventions to promote healthy behaviors in pediatric and adolescent populations: implications for clinical practice and research. Worldviews Evidence-Based Nurs 2012;9(2):66–77.

32. Sharifi M, Dryden EM, Horan CM, et al. Leveraging text messaging and mobile technology to support pediatric obesity-related behavior change: a qualitative study using parent focus groups and interviews. J Med Internet Res 2013;15(12):e272.

33. Dudas RA, Pumilia JN, Crocetti M. Pediatric caregiver attitudes and technologic readiness toward electronic follow-up communication in an urban community emergency department. Telemed J E Health 2013;19(6):493–6.

34. Ridings LE, Anton MT, Winkelmann J, et al. Trauma resilience and recovery program: addressing mental health in pediatric trauma centers. J Pediatr Psychol 2019;44(9):1046–56.

35. Taylor SL, Meyer JM, Munoz-Abraham AS, et al. Standardized text messages improve 30-day patient follow-up for ACS pediatric NSQIP cases. Pediatr Surg Int 2019;35(4):523–7.

36. Newton L, Sulman C. Use of text messaging to improve patient experience and communication with pediatric tonsillectomy patients. Int J Pediatr Otorhinolaryngol 2018;113:213–7.
37. Gahleitner F, Legg J, Holland E, et al. The validity and acceptability of a text-based monitoring system for pediatric asthma studies. Pediatr pulmonology 2016;51(1):5–12.
38. Stephens TN, Joerin A, Rauws M, et al. Feasibility of pediatric obesity and prediabetes treatment support through Tess, the AI behavioral coaching chatbot. Translational behavioral medicine 2019;9(3):440–7.
39. Hofstetter AM, Vargas CY, Camargo S, et al. Impacting delayed pediatric influenza vaccination: a randomized controlled trial of text message reminders. Am J Prev Med 2015;48(4):392–401.
40. Sloand E, VanGraafeiland B, Holm A, et al. Text message quality improvement project for influenza vaccine in a low-resource largely Latino pediatric population. J Healthc Qual 2019;41(6):362–8.
41. Stockwell MS, Kharbanda EO, Martinez RA, et al. Effect of a text messaging intervention on influenza vaccination in an urban, low-income pediatric and adolescent population: a randomized controlled trial. JAMA 2012;307(16):1702–8.
42. Wang C-s, Troost JP, Greenbaum LA, et al. Text messaging for disease monitoring in childhood nephrotic syndrome. Kidney Int Rep 2019;4(8):1066–74.
43. Mellor X, Buczek MJ, Adams AJ, et al. Collection of common knee patient-reported outcome instruments by automated mobile phone text messaging in pediatric sports medicine. J Pediatr Orthop 2020;40(2):e91–5.
44. Flores-Fenlon N, Song AY, Yeh A, et al. Smartphones and text messaging are associated with higher parent quality of life scores and enrollment in early intervention after NICU discharge. Clin Pediatr 2019;58(8):903–11.
45. Zhao Y, Zhu X, Pérez AE, et al. MHealth approach to promote oral HIV self-testing among men who have sex with men in China: a qualitative description. BMC Public Health 2018;18(1):1146.
46. Storck L. Policy statement: texting in health care. On Line J Nurs Inform 2017;21(1).
47. Kuhlmann S, Ahlers-Schmidt CR, Steinberger E. TXT@ WORK: pediatric hospitalists and text messaging. Telemed J E Health 2014;20(7):647–52.
48. Khorsand K, Sidbury R. The shadow clinic: emails, "curbsides," and "quick peeks" in pediatric dermatology. Pediatr Dermatol 2019;36(5):607–10.
49. Drolet BC, Marwaha JS, Hyatt B, et al. Electronic communication of protected health information: privacy, security, and HIPAA compliance. J Hand Surg 2017;42(6):411–6.

Implementing Telehealth in Pediatric Asthma

Tamara T. Perry, MD[a,b,*], Callie A. Margiotta, BS[b]

KEYWORDS

• Telemedicine • Asthma • Pediatrics

KEY POINTS

- Telemedicine can be used to deliver recommended asthma care in regions with inadequate access to specialists.
- Telemedicine can be used for pediatric asthma care to reduce travel burden for rural patients and families.
- Telemedicine can be used to reach patients in a variety of settings, including school-based and community settings.

PROBLEM TO BE SOLVED BY TELEMEDICINE

Asthma is one of the most frequent causes of pediatric health care use, with more than 1.8 million emergency department (ED) visits annually among children, and more than 13.8 million school days missed annually because of follow-up doctors' visits, acute illness, or uncontrolled symptoms.[1,2] Risk factors for poor asthma outcomes include increased exposure to environmental triggers,[3] financial barriers,[4] and reduced social support.[5] Uncontrolled asthma can lead to significant financial and social strain caused by costs associated with acute health care use[6]; time away from work for caregivers[7]; and travel, especially among patients living in rural regions who have to drive long distances to see their nearest asthma specialist.[8] Prior research has shown that guidelines-based care is more likely when asthma care is managed by a specialist,[9] and better outcomes are associated with guidelines-based care.[10] However, patients with the greatest need for asthma specialists often live in underserved areas, such as rural and low-income communities, where few asthma specialists exist.[11] Telemedicine should be used to remove or significantly reduce barriers to specialty care.

[a] Department of Pediatrics, University of Arkansas for Medical Sciences, 4301 West Markham Street, Little Rock, AR 72205, USA; [b] Arkansas Children's Research Institute, 13 Children's Way, Slot 512-13, Little Rock, AR 72202, USA
* Corresponding author. Department of Pediatrics, Allergy and Immunology Division, University of Arkansas for Medical Sciences, 13 Children's Way, Slot 512-13, Little Rock, AR 72202.
E-mail address: perrytamarat@uams.edu

Pediatr Clin N Am 67 (2020) 623–627
https://doi.org/10.1016/j.pcl.2020.04.003
0031-3955/20/© 2020 Elsevier Inc. All rights reserved.

CAN TELEMEDICINE BE USED TO IMPROVE ASTHMA CARE?

Asthma is a chronic condition with variability in symptoms over time caused by underlying severity, medication adherence, trigger exposure, and seasonal changes. National asthma guidelines recommend targeted asthma education and regular follow-up care as key aspects for monitoring disease control and asthma management.[10]

Because children spend most of their waking hours at school, prior investigations have assessed the use of school-based telemedicine (SBTM) interventions to improve asthma outcomes for underserved populations.[12] Perry and colleagues[13] implemented a randomized controlled trial in the rural Delta region of Arkansas to assess the effectiveness of an SBTM asthma education program compared with usual care among children enrolled in public schools. There was evidence of behavior change for intervention participants, with improvement in reported use of asthma medications and peak flow meter monitoring. However, no significant differences in the number of symptom-free-days (SFDs), compared with baseline, were found for either group. Investigators concluded that tele-education alone was insufficient to overcome the significant baseline morbidity among the study population.[13] Halterman and colleagues[14] implemented a comprehensive SBTM intervention that included directly observed therapy for daily preventive asthma medications as well as telemedicine follow-up care visits with the child's primary care provider. Children in the intervention group had more SFDs and reduced acute health care use compared with an enhanced usual-care group. Other investigators have proved feasibility for implementing SBTM interventions as well as their effectiveness in improving asthma outcomes, such as reduction in ED visits and improved quality of life.[15,16]

Asthma guidelines recommend that changes in medication therapy be guided by patient-reported symptoms and/or objective findings, such as lung function testing (or spirometry).[10] Spirometry with highly trained asthma specialists and respiratory therapists is particularly important among pediatric patients, who may need specific coaching and other techniques geared for children. For patients living in regions with poor access to specialty care, remote spirometry via telemedicine allows guidelines-based recommendations to monitor lung function. Berlinski and colleagues[17] reported the successful implementation of remote spirometry in rural settings with no adverse events and rates of interpretable spirometry data resembling rates of in-person spirometry.

Asthma guidelines address the importance of self-management through the use of a personalized asthma action plan[10] (AAP). Traditional paper AAPs are static, lack patient engagement,[18] and require patients to keep track of a paper document. To address these concerns, Perry and colleagues[19] implemented a randomized trial to compare the use and effectiveness of an interactive smartphone-based AAP with paper AAP among teens, a group at risk for poor asthma outcomes. Patients in the intervention group accessed their smartphone AAP more times per week compared with the paper AAP group. Intervention subjects with uncontrolled asthma at baseline showed improved Asthma Control Test scores after using the smartphone AAP for 6 months, whereas no improvements were seen in the control group. Findings suggest smartphone AAPs are a feasible method for improving self-management and asthma outcomes in this hard-to-reach pediatric population.

DIFFICULTIES AND BARRIERS TO IMPLEMENTATION OF TELEMEDICINE
Funding and Reimbursement

Financial sustainability is a significant barrier to establishing as well as maintaining a telemedicine program. The cost of technology proves to be a deciding factor, because of the need for significant investment in infrastructure when implementing telemedicine programs. Comprehensive telemedicine carts cost $10,000 to $35,000 for a single site,[20] plus there may be additional costs associated with the purchase of Health Insurance Portability and Accountability Act–compliant software. For rural telemedicine sites, high-speed Internet capabilities may be another added expense because these sites often lack the bandwidth to support the high-quality videoconferencing necessary for satisfactory telemedicine visits.[21]

In a national survey of pediatric telemedicine programs, lack of financial reimbursement is also cited as a main barrier to implementing telemedicine.[20] Parity in coverage and reimbursement is not currently federally mandated, and each state does not define and regulate telehealth in the same way, so states differ in the extent to which insurers reimburse.[22] To receive universal acceptance, there is a need for consistent state policy backing and increased government stakeholder support for implementing telemedicine programs.

Provider licensure and uptake

Another barrier includes licensure for physicians who want to provide remote care for patients across state lines. Regulations require provider licensure in the state of the originating site (patient's location), limiting providers' ability to see patients outside their home states, unless they are licensed in multiple states. The Interstate Medical Licensure Compact (IMLC) offers an expedited pathway for multistate licensure; however, IMLC is not available in all states. Another significant barrier to telemedicine is provider readiness and acceptability. Some providers are hesitant to implement telemedicine because of concerns that technology depersonalizes the patient-physician relationship.[23] However, current literature supports the use of telemedicine, with reports of high patient satisfaction because of the convenience, which enhances providers' ability to reach their patients.[8,24] Physicians need proper training to use the software and equipment because, with technology, there is always a possibility for technological glitches or lags that can further complicate the physician and patient experience. Physicians also must have a backup plan if the connection is lost as well as needing to set enough time before each visit to run tests, making sure there are no connectivity issues.[8] These extra steps for providing care outside of the traditional clinic setting can seem daunting if physicians are not properly informed of the added benefits of telemedicine. The health care industry is beginning to adapt to the ever-changing technological environment, albeit at a slower rate than technology is advancing. In light of this, physicians and the health care community should embrace these advances and integrate telemedicine into the medical school curriculum.

POTENTIAL FOR COST SAVINGS

Asthma is the third leading cause of hospitalizations in children younger than 15 years,[25] resulting in a significant health care cost burden. Acute health care use is dramatically reduced or avoided through proper asthma management.[26] Because outpatient care generally costs less for insurance companies than hospital-based inpatient care, conducting follow-up visits via telemedicine is a viable option to provide accessible and cost-effective preventive care. Bian and colleagues[15] report on the successful implementation of school-based telemedicine clinics that allowed students who needed immediate care during school hours to see pediatric clinicians. Clinicians were able to provide prompt clinical services to children as well as school nurse education on the proper administration of asthma medications. Investigators reported a 21% reduction in ED visits among the subsample of children with asthma.

According to a 2016 study, no-show rates of in-person visits in the United States exceed 20%.[27] Telemedicine can relieve this burden by making follow-up care more accessible. Portnoy and colleagues[28] reported that patients enrolled in telemedicine visits were more likely to complete all 3 of their follow-up asthma visits compared with usual in-person visits. This finding further encourages health care cost-saving opportunities by decreasing no-show rates and allowing specialists to see more patients.

SUMMARY

The nature of chronic disease management such as asthma in children calls for collaboration between patients, parents, educators, and physicians. Telemedicine has the potential to reach patients in a variety of settings, including school-based and community settings, thus providing more accessible care to patients who are at the highest risk. Inadequate access to specialists and travel burden for patients and families can lead to school/work absenteeism and poor compliance with treatment plans. Increased rates of cancellations and no-shows can lead to uncontrolled asthma outcomes requiring hospitalizations and acute health care use. Telemedicine provides an avenue for increasing convenient access to specialty care, leading to increased compliance with treatment plans. Current literature suggests that telemedicine is comparable with in-person asthma care. However, with continued implementation of larger-scale research designs, there is a call to further prove that these various telehealth models are not only equally effective but can improve patient satisfaction and chronic disease control long term. Technological advancements continue to increase the scope that medical practices reach, proving telemedicine to be beneficial for patients, providers, health care companies, and insurers. With the climate of the health care system and the difficulties clinicians now face, it is vital for telemedicine to be used as a solution to deliver convenient patient care to all.

DISCLOSURE

The authors have nothing to disclose.

REFERENCES

1. Zahran HS, Bailey CM, Damon SA, et al. Vital signs: asthma in children - United States, 2001-2016. MMWR Morb Mortal Wkly Rep 2018;67:149–55.
2. Johnson LH, Chambers P, Dexheimer JW. Asthma-related emergency department use: current perspectives. Open Access Emerg Med 2016;8:47–55.
3. Coleman AT, Rettiganti M, Bai S, et al. Mouse and cockroach exposure in rural Arkansas Delta region homes. Ann Allergy Asthma Immunol 2014;112:256–60.
4. Beck AF, Huang B, Simmons JM, et al. Role of financial and social hardships in asthma racial disparities. Pediatrics 2014;133:431–9.
5. Williams DR, Sternthal M, Wright RJ. Social determinants: taking the social context of asthma seriously. Pediatrics 2009;123(Suppl 3):S174–84.
6. Nurmagambetov T, Kuwahara R, Garbe P. The economic burden of asthma in the United States, 2008-2013. Ann Am Thorac Soc 2018;15:348–56.
7. Dean BB, Calimlim BM, Kindermann SL, et al. The impact of uncontrolled asthma on absenteeism and health-related quality of life. J Asthma 2009;46:861–6.
8. Taylor L, Waller M, Portnoy JM. Telemedicine for allergy services to rural communities. J Allergy Clin Immunol Pract 2019;7(8):2554–9.
9. Diette GB, Skinner EA, Nguyen TT, et al. Comparison of quality of care by specialist and generalist physicians as usual source of asthma care for children. Pediatrics 2001;108:432–7.

10. National asthma education and prevention program expert panel report 3: guidelines for the Diagnosis and Management of Asthma. National Heart Lung and Blood Institute; 2007. NIH Publication No. 07-4051. 2012.
11. Ownby DR. Asthma in rural America. Ann Allergy Asthma Immunol 2005;95: S17–22.
12. Perry TT, Turner JH. School-based telemedicine for asthma management. J Allergy Clin Immunol Pract 2019;7:2524–32.
13. Perry TT, Halterman JS, Brown RH, et al. Results of an asthma education program delivered via telemedicine in rural schools. Ann Allergy Asthma Immunol 2018; 120:401–8.
14. Halterman JS, Fagnano M, Tajon RS, et al. Effect of the school-based telemedicine enhanced asthma management (SB-TEAM) program on asthma morbidity: a randomized clinical trial. JAMA Pediatr 2018;172:e174938.
15. Bian J, Cristaldi KK, Summer AP, et al. Association of a school-based, asthma-focused telehealth program with emergency department visits among children enrolled in South Carolina Medicaid. JAMA Pediatr 2019. https://doi.org/10.1001/jamapediatrics.2019.3073.
16. Romano MJ, Hernandez J, Gaylor A, et al. Improvement in asthma symptoms and quality of life in pediatric patients through specialty care delivered via telemedicine. Telemed J E Health 2001;7:281–6.
17. Berlinski A, Chervinskiy SK, Simmons AL, et al. Delivery of high-quality pediatric spirometry in rural communities: A novel use for telemedicine. J Allergy Clin Immunol Pract 2018;6:1042–4.
18. Hynes L, Durkin K, Williford DN, et al. Comparing written versus pictorial asthma action plans to improve asthma management and health outcomes among children and adolescents: protocol of a pilot and feasibility randomized controlled trial. JMIR Res Protoc 2019;8:e11733.
19. Perry TT, Marshall A, Berlinski A, et al. Smartphone-based vs paper-based asthma action plans for adolescents. Ann Allergy Asthma Immunol 2017;118: 298–303.
20. Olson CA, McSwain SD, Curfman AL, et al. The current pediatric telehealth landscape. Pediatrics 2018;141 [pii:e20172334].
21. Scott Kruse C, Karem P, Shifflett K, et al. Evaluating barriers to adopting telemedicine worldwide: A systematic review. J Telemed Telecare 2018;24:4–12.
22. Available at: https://www.cchpca.org/sites/default/files/2019-05/cchp_report_MASTER_spring_2019_FINAL.pdf. Accessed October 1, 2019.
23. Elliott T, Shih J, Dinakar C, et al. American College of Allergy, Asthma & Immunology position paper on the use of telemedicine for allergists. Ann Allergy Asthma Immunol 2017;119:512–7.
24. Utidjian L, Abramson E. Pediatric telehealth: opportunities and challenges. Pediatr Clin North Am 2016;63:367–78.
25. Available at: https://www.epa.gov/sites/production/files/2016-05/documents/asthma_fact_sheet_english_05_2016.pdf. Accessed October 1, 2019.
26. Rangachari P. A framework for measuring self-management effectiveness and health care use among pediatric asthma patients and families. J Asthma Allergy 2017;10:111–22.
27. Kheirkhah P, Feng Q, Travis LM, et al. Prevalence, predictors and economic consequences of no-shows. BMC Health Serv Res 2016;16:13.
28. Portnoy JM, Waller M, De Lurgio S, et al. Telemedicine is as effective as in-person visits for patients with asthma. Ann Allergy Asthma Immunol 2016;117:241–5.

A Multimodal Telehealth Strategy to Improve Pediatric Epilepsy Care

Madeline H. Niemann, BA[a], Manuel C. Alvarado, BS[a,b],
Cristina Camayd-Muñoz, MS[a], Rinat R. Jonas, MD[a],
Jodi K. Wenger, MD[a,c], Laurie M. Douglass, MD[a,*]

KEYWORDS

- Epilepsy • Seizures • Complex care • Telehealth • Telemedicine
- Patient-centered medical home

KEY POINTS

- Telehealth tools can improve communication between providers, patients, family members, and community systems involved in complex care management.
- Telehealth tools can be particularly useful in the context of populations experiencing health care disparities, because telemedicine visits may reduce costs for patients and boost appointment attendance. Teens and youth may also be particularly well served by telehealth because of generational communication preferences.
- New telehealth projects should expect to include patient and family perspectives, a strong network of internal and community supports, and specific workflows that reduce click fatigue.
- For telehealth interventions to become sustainable, there must be additional support at the state level to expand reimbursement policies for providers.

INTRODUCTION

The Telehealth Epilepsy Care Collaborative (TECC) is a network of medical providers, public health researchers, patients, and families committed to improving care for children and youth with epilepsy (CYE) through technology. TECC emphasizes serving

Funding: Funding for this project comes from the Maternal and Child Health Bureau within the Health Resources and Services Administration, and is administered by the American Academy of Pediatrics.
[a] Division of Pediatric Neurology, Departments of Pediatrics and Neurology, Boston Medical Center, 801 Albany St, Suite 1028N, Boston, MA 02119, USA; [b] Boston University School of Public Health, Boston, MA, USA; [c] Division of Pediatrics, Boston Medical Center, Boston, MA, USA
* Corresponding author. Division of Pediatric Neurology, Departments of Pediatrics and Neurology, Boston Medical Center, 801 Albany St, Suite 1028N, Boston, MA 02119.
E-mail address: Laurie.Douglass@bmc.org

Pediatr Clin N Am 67 (2020) 629–634
https://doi.org/10.1016/j.pcl.2020.04.004
0031-3955/20/© 2020 Elsevier Inc. All rights reserved.

CYE affected by health care disparities and geographic barriers. Interventions are spread between Boston Medical Center (BMC) and 11 other pediatric practices, 10 located in allied community health care centers within Massachusetts. Using funds provided through the Maternal and Child Health Bureau at the Health Resources and Service Administration, TECC designed a unique, multimodal telehealth platform to improve care access and care coordination for CYE in 2016.

Epilepsy as a Model of Complex Care Management

Epilepsy is both common and chronic, costing Americans nearly $10 billion in annual treatment expenses.[1] At least 1 in 10 individuals experiences a seizure in their lifetimes, and 1 in 26 develop epilepsy,[2] making affordable and accessible seizure management essential for many. In addition, more than 50% of CYE have comorbid behavioral, learning, or psychiatric comorbidities, and so often navigate between multiple health care providers.[3–5] Pediatric epilepsy care may serve as a model for any patient with complex care needs, or any provider undertaking significant care coordination efforts.

Families and other caregivers provide a crucial link between the health care system and the community, but this link is underused. Patient portals housed within electronic medical record systems have made it easier for patients to connect with their providers, but these systems often exclude outside health care providers such as school nurses, therapists, and home services, making care coordination a challenge across health and education systems.

Barriers to Care for Children and Youth with Epilepsy at Boston Medical Center

Each year, TECC providers care for more than 650 CYE in the division of pediatric neurology at BMC. Almost 60% of BMC's patient population live in underserved communities and are likely to receive their primary care at neighborhood health centers. In Massachusetts, 90% of health center patients have incomes less than 200% of the federal poverty level and 63% belong to an ethnic or racial minority group.[6] This finding is significant, because children receiving public health insurance have an increased burden of epilepsy but less consistent access to specialty care.[7] Despite these challenges, TECC found that more than 90% of clinic patients have reliable access to the Internet and a video call–enabled device from home.[8]

A Multimodal Strategy for Complex Care

In order to ease care coordination and overcome persistent health care barriers, TECC developed the virtual patient-centered medical home (VPCMH), which applies the foundations of a traditional patient-centered medical home to a Health Insurance Portability and Accountability Act (HIPAA)–secure, cloud-based platform.[9]

The VPCMH improves communication between the entire care team and patient. It overcomes the barrier of electronic medical record siloes, saves time often wasted by telephone tag, ensures patient privacy, and can connect the entire care team to the patient regardless of location. The VPCMH is accessible by any Internet-enabled device and new members are invited over e-mail. Patients and parents can grant access to any member of their care team to the VPCMH platform, while also being able to restrict access to sections containing sensitive information. Other functions of the VPCMH include (1) developing and sharing a treatment and seizure action plan, (2) goal setting, (3) task reminders, (4) logging key medical events such as seizures, (5) collecting medical assessments, and (6) sharing targeted education resources. Teens with epilepsy who are expected to become independent are also provided with a transition plan and have the option to receive one-on-one self-management mentoring over the platform.

Figs. 1–3 show a standard VPCMH profile, which is coded and managed by a third party health technology company, ACT.md.

Treating Epilepsy over Video Call

In addition to the telehealth features mentioned earlier, the VPCMH facilitates video call appointments (telemedicine) and secure messaging features. These features reduce the need for patients to traverse barriers and pay additional service fees to receive care.

For patients with known epilepsy, there are many needs that can be met via video calling. Clinicians can provide care into the primary care provider's office and assist with triage. They can also provide care into the home, school, or workplace, thereby minimizing lost work and school days. Video calling has allowed clinicians to view patients after starting new medications and identify side-effects. It is also a wonderful tool for counseling patients about medications and assessing the patient/family understanding of the treatment plan. For children with neurodevelopmental disabilities, telemedicine can reduce patient/family stress and allow the provider to observe the patient within the home or school environment. The authors have used video calling for groups, such as multidisciplinary meetings, online support groups, and a family advisory board.

Lessons Learned on Implementation

- Teens and young adults may be particularly well suited for telehealth services. Adolescents now prefer technology to face-to-face encounters. They rely on texting, social media apps, and video chats.[10] CYE that never reached out to their care teams via phone are now reaching out via texting and video calling.
- New telehealth initiatives require significant supports and teamwork. Between 2016 and 2019, TECC staff trained more than 71 community volunteers and 3 full-time AmeriCorps VISTAs (Volunteers in Service to America) to develop this

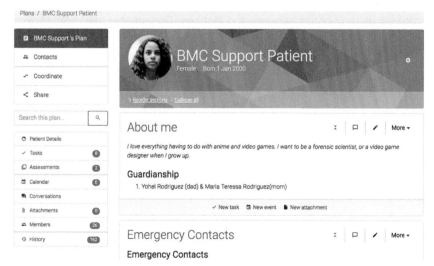

Fig. 1. Patient profiles resemble social media pages.

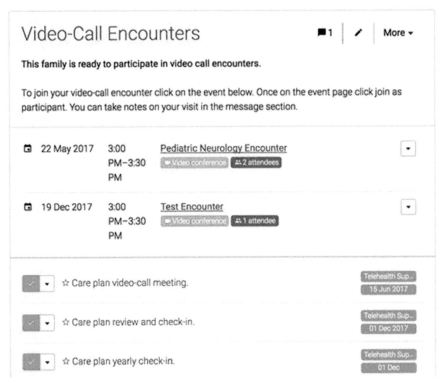

Fig. 2. Patients can meet with their providers for HIPAA-secure video call appointments using their VPCMH portals.

model at BMC. A comparable, multimodal telehealth project would be best facilitated by a paid staff member, or several.

- Patients should be involved in the design of telehealth platforms. A family advisory board of diverse patients and caregivers helped design the VPCMH, which allowed us to prioritize services and features. Comparable telehealth projects

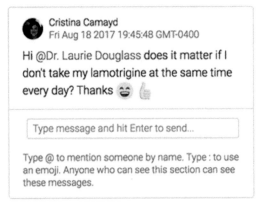

Fig. 3. A conversations feature lets patients and caregivers reach providers with nonurgent questions.

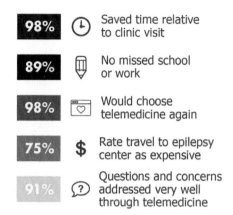

98%	🕐	Saved time relative to clinic visit
89%	✏️	No missed school or work
98%	🖥️	Would choose telemedicine again
75%	$	Rate travel to epilepsy center as expensive
91%	❓	Questions and concerns addressed very well through telemedicine

No patients/families reported audio or visual disturbances.
Families avoided an average travel time of 1.5 h
to the epilepsy center. (n = 57)

Fig. 4. Telemedicine satisfaction survey results.

should include explicit budgeting measures that incentivize, compensate, and make diverse patient feedback viable throughout each stage of development.

- Telehealth interventions must ease workflows for everyone involved. New telehealth projects must clearly ease already strenuous workflows for providers. Patients must also believe that the telehealth platform makes their lives easier. So-called click fatigue is enduring in portable medical records.[11]

Supportive Data

Between 2016 and 2019, TECC provided 350 unique patients with a VPCMH and facilitated 139 telemedicine visits. Posttelemedicine patient/family surveys have been positive (**Fig. 4**). The no-show rate for visits with epilepsy specialists was halved, a reduction from 15% for in-person visits to 7% using telemedicine; revenue loss was likewise halved. These results suggest that telemedicine is saving a vulnerable population missed wages, transportation costs, and additional clinic fees while enabling more frequent and personalized care.

Next Steps

TECC was fortunate to be refunded through the Maternal and Child Health Bureau at the Health Resources and Service Administration through 2023. The next steps that will help achieve the network's goal of improving access to quality of care using telehealth include (1) completion of a Spanish VPCMH template; (2) collaboration with additional community partners and support organizations, such as the Epilepsy Foundation of New England; and (3) analyzing and sharing our outcome data to inform health care policies regarding telehealth and telemedicine reimbursement in Massachusetts.

DISCLOSURE

The VPCMH is coded and maintained by the health technology company, ACT.md. The project did not receive funding from ACT.md. The authors have no conflicts to disclose.

REFERENCES

1. Yoon D, Frick KD, Carr DA, et al. Economic impact of epilepsy in the United States. Epilepsia 2009;50(10):2186–91.
2. Hesdorffer DC, Logroscino G, Benn EKT, et al. Estimating risk for developing epilepsy: a population-based study in Rochester, Minnesota. Neurology 2011; 76(1):23–7.
3. Wagner JL, Wilson DA, Smith G, et al. Neurodevelopmental and mental health comorbidities in children and adolescents with epilepsy and migraine: a response to identified research gaps. Dev Med Child Neurol 2015;57(1):45–52.
4. Russ SA, Larson K, Halfon N. A national profile of childhood epilepsy and seizure disorder. Pediatrics 2012;129(2):256–64.
5. Jensen FE. Epilepsy as a spectrum disorder: Implications from novel clinical and basic neuroscience. Epilepsia 2011;52(Suppl 1):1–6.
6. A Novel Parent Questionnaire for the Detection of Seizures in Children - Pediatric Neurology. Available at: https://www.pedneur.com/article/S0887-8994(15)00472-5/fulltext. Accessed September 30, 2019.
7. Schiltz NK, Koroukian SM, Singer ME, et al. Disparities In Access To Specialized Epilepsy Care. Epilepsy Res 2013;107. https://doi.org/10.1016/j.eplepsyres.2013.08.003.
8. Camayd-Muñoz C, Miller EL, Rollins JV et al. Capability of implementing telehealth in a pediatric neurology population with high health disparities. Poster presented at: Child Neurology Society Meeting. Kansas City, MO, October 4–7, 2017.
9. Defining the Virtual Patient-Centered Medical Home - Nuss S, Camayd-Muñoz C, Jonas R, et al. 2018. Available at: https://journals.sagepub.com/doi/10.1177/0009922818793355. Accessed September 30, 2019.
10. Teens Are Over Face-to-Face Communication, Study Says | Time. Available at: https://time.com/5390435/teen-social-media-usage/. Accessed September 30, 2019.
11. Rodriguez Torres Y, Huang J, Mihlstin M, et al. The effect of electronic health record software design on resident documentation and compliance with evidence-based medicine. PLoS One 2017;12(9):e0185052.

Telehealth in Pediatric Heart Transplant Patients

Exercise, Nutrition, and Parental Imaging

Angela C. Chen, BS, Elif Seda Selamet Tierney, MD*

KEYWORDS

- Telehealth • Echocardiography • Pediatrics • Heart Transplant • Home-monitoring
- Live-Video Conferencing

KEY POINTS

- Telehealth is a promising new tool in medicine that has changed the landscape of medical care.
- The benefits of telehealth technology are immense, including improved access to care and potential savings in monetary and opportunity costs.
- Current challenges of incorporating telehealth services into regular clinical care include licensure and regulatory barriers, difficulty obtaining insurance reimbursements, and high costs of setting up successful telehealth infrastructures.
- These challenges threaten telehealth's future scalability and expansion to reach all patients in need.

INTRODUCTION

Telehealth is a promising new tool in medicine that has changed the landscape of medical care. A 2018 database of 52 pediatric telehealth programs shows that neurology, psychiatry, neonatology, critical care, and cardiology are among the top 5 specialties offering telehealth services.[1] Telehealth intervention programs have also been successfully used to manage pediatric diabetes and obesity.[2,3] The benefits of telehealth technology are immense, including improved access to care and potential savings in monetary and opportunity costs.[4,5] Patients in rural communities without nearby specialized centers are able to see experts without extensive travel. In addition, patients who have difficulty scheduling clinic visits because of school or work obligations are

Funding: Cardiovascular Institute Seed Grant, Stanford University; American Heart Association Grant-in-Aid Grant number: 15GRNT25680030; and American Council on Exercise.

Division of Pediatric Cardiology, Department of Pediatrics, Stanford University Medical Center, Palo Alto, CA, USA

* Corresponding author. Heart Center, Stanford Children Health, Stanford University, 750 Welch Road, Suite 325, Mail Code 5721, Palo Alto, CA 94304.

E-mail address: tierneys@stanford.edu

given more flexibility and the ability to schedule home appointments. Current challenges of incorporating telehealth services into regular clinical care include licensure and regulatory barriers, difficulty obtaining insurance reimbursements, and high costs of setting up successful telehealth infrastructures.[1,6] These challenges threaten telehealth's future scalability and expansion to reach all patients in need.

In our center at Lucile Packard Children's Hospital, Stanford University, we have piloted the use of telehealth in the care of pediatric heart transplant patients. These patients are ideal candidates for telehealth interventions because the patients and their families are already heavily burdened with the frequency of clinic follow-up visits as part of their long-term care after transplant. Pediatric heart transplant patients followed in our center also often live far from hospitals with pediatric echocardiographic (echo) imaging capacity, resulting in urgent/emergent transfers to specialized institutions if there is any concern about their cardiac conditions. Expensive and time-consuming transportation to overcome these geographic boundaries inevitably interferes with health care access and increases emotional and financial stress. In addition, heart transplant recipients have increased cardiovascular risk profiles that contribute to their long-term mortality and morbidity. Current clinical focus has been on pharmacologic management, without much emphasis on routine exercise or healthy nutrition as part of clinical care. Even though an on-site exercise program could improve cardiovascular health in these patients, on-site exercise and diet interventions in children and adolescents report low adherence, often because of barriers such as distance to site, transportation difficulties, and school or work obligations (**Fig. 1**).[7]

The 2 following telehealth studies in our pediatric heart transplant patients address some of these issues:

Parental Acquisition of Echocardiographic Images in Pediatric Heart Transplant Patients Using a Hand-Held Device: A Pilot Telehealth Study

We evaluated the feasibility of parental acquisition of echo images to assess left ventricular systolic function in pediatric heart transplant patients (**Fig. 2**).[8]

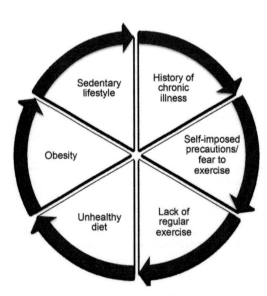

Fig. 1. Barriers to a heart-healthy lifestyle in pediatric heart transplant patients.

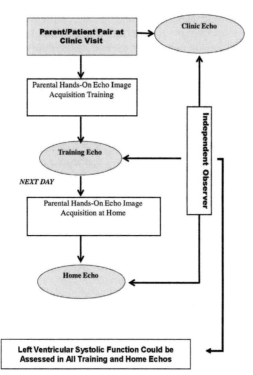

Fig. 2. Parental home echo acquisition in pediatric heart transplant patients. (*From* Dykes JC, Kipps AK, Chen A, et al. Parental acquisition of echocardiographic images in pediatric heart transplant patients using a handheld device: a pilot telehealth study. J Am Soc Echocardiogr. 2019;32:405; with permission.)

Echocardiography and telemedicine have already been widely implemented where a sonographer or specialized provider obtains ultrasonography images from a patient and then transmits them to an off-site cardiologist.[6] This study examined whether parents, rather than experienced professionals, could be trained to obtain echo images of their children. After a routine clinic visit, a pediatric cardiologist specialized in imaging led a 1-hour training session to teach parents of heart transplant patients to acquire images in parasternal short-axis and apical views using a hand-held echo device. Parents were instructed to reimage their children at home the following day with the same device. Home, clinical, and training echos were reviewed by a pediatric cardiologist. All parents were able to acquire home images adequate for qualitative assessment of left ventricular systolic function. Most parents reported that they felt at least moderately comfortable using the device. Furthermore, multiple parents expressed sentiments of empowerment to contribute to their children's care.

These results are encouraging; however, it is conceivable that parents of heart transplant patients are a highly motivated group who may feel empowered having an additional tool to assist in their children's care. Another perspective could be that parents of children with transplanted hearts or decreased left ventricular systolic function may be under a great deal of stress and learning a new technique to acquire echo images on their children may further compound that stress. Thus, not every parent might be well-suited for this role in their children's care.

The authors believe that using telehealth to complement clinic-based long-term echo surveillance of heart transplant patients could be an important new tool to allow parental home acquisition of echo images and subsequent immediate qualitative assessment of left ventricular systolic function in pediatric heart transplant patients after transmission to interpreting physicians. However, quantitative assessment of left ventricular systolic function and the retention of the skillset 1 year later without additional training were suboptimal, indicating the need for additional training/refresher sessions.

Future steps should explore the efficacy of an echo training program with follow-up refresher sessions for retention of the imaging skill set. In addition, a secure, Health Insurance Portability and Accountability Act (HIPAA)–compliant infrastructure for transmission of the images for immediate remote assessment is imperative for clinical use of home echos. Physician and patient location are also important to note because physicians may need to be licensed and registered in the state in which the patient is located.[1,6] This requirement could be a significant barrier to expanding a similar program nationally. Although the initial costs of both physician time to train parents and the portable echo machines are high, over the lifespans of heart transplant patients, costs saved from unnecessary emergency care, travel, and clinical echos are hypothesized to more than offset the initial setup costs.

Healthy Hearts via Live-Video Conferencing: an Exercise and Diet Intervention in Pediatric Heart Transplant Patients

Our team conducted a supervised exercise and diet program delivered via live-video conferencing in pediatric heart transplant patients.[9] Patients in this telehealth lifestyle program were given tablets to use at home. They exercised with a trainer 3 times a week and met with a nutrition counselor once a week in the first 12 to 16 weeks, all in real time. After completion of this intense phase, patients entered a maintenance phase where they exercised with a trainer only once a week and continued to meet with the nutrition counselor once a week for an additional 12 to 16 weeks. During this phase, patients were instructed to exercise on their own at least twice a week. Adherence rates to both the exercise and nutrition sessions were greater than 80%, strikingly higher than what has been reported in prior on-site pediatric intervention studies (<50%, and as low as 10%).[7] Parents reported the ease of scheduling sessions at home based on their availability as the main contributor to high attendance rates. Patients in our live video–supervised lifestyle intervention showed significant improvement in Vo_2 max (maximum oxygen consumption) and percent predicted Vo_2 max, which were sustained even after the maintenance phase.

There were a few difficulties and limitations with the telehealth delivery of our exercise and nutrition lifestyle program. The program required significant time investment from the study team to set up the tablets for individual use. Sessions were scheduled by a weekly phone call or text, but we often had to remind patients of their sessions if they were not logged in within 5 minutes of their scheduled start times.

Parental influence was critical in each patient's overall engagement with the study. Patients whose parents were more involved in scheduling and present for exercise and nutrition sessions were more likely to have consistent participation, although we did not collect these data quantitatively. An HIPAA-compliant online scheduler, where participants could choose their weekly sessions from predetermined time slots and have automatic reminders sent, could reduce unnecessary time and costs spent reminding participants of their individual sessions.

The known benefits of exercise on cardiovascular health and the demonstrated feasibility of this intervention suggest our telehealth approach might have important implications for the long-term health and survival of pediatric heart transplant patients. The potential health care and opportunity cost savings from this telehealth preventive lifestyle intervention are high. Patients with improved capacity may have fewer complications from their transplants, requiring fewer emergency room visits and pharmacologic interventions. In addition, the at-home delivery of the program reduces time and costs associated with traveling to clinic-based exercise and nutrition programs. The next steps should be to test the feasibility of group-based telehealth interventions to increase scalability and further reduce costs and assess the impact of regular exercise on outcomes in this population.

SUMMARY

Our studies in the pediatric heart transplant population have shown that parental home echo acquisition using a hand-held echo device is feasible and adequate for remote qualitative assessment of left ventricular systolic function and that telehealth can be used to successfully deliver a lifestyle intervention. The benefits of both of these studies can be applied to other pediatric populations with chronic medical conditions; however, further research is needed to evaluate the clinical settings in which telehealth would be useful to clinicians, patients, and parents, and what its impact would be to patient care and resource use.

DISCLOSURE

The authors have nothing to disclose.

REFERENCES

1. Olson CA, McSwain SD, Curfman AL, et al. The current pediatric telehealth landscape. Pediatrics 2018;141 [pii:e20172334].
2. Guttmann-Bauman I, Kono J, Lin AL, et al. Use of telehealth videoconferencing in pediatric type 1 diabetes in Oregon. Telemed J E Health 2018;24:86–8.
3. Nourse SE, Olson I, Popat RA, et al. Live video diet and exercise intervention in overweight and obese youth: adherence and cardiovascular health. J Pediatr 2015;167:533–539 e1.
4. Lindgren S, Wacker D, Suess A, et al. Telehealth and autism: treating challenging behavior at lower cost. Pediatrics 2016;137(Suppl 2):S167–75.
5. Jue JS, Spector SA, Spector SA. Telemedicine broadening access to care for complex cases. J Surg Res 2017;220:164–70.
6. Satou GM, Rheuban K, Alverson D, et al. Telemedicine in pediatric cardiology: a scientific statement from the American Heart Association. Circulation 2017;135: e648–78.
7. Hampl S, Paves H, Laubscher K, et al. Patient engagement and attrition in pediatric obesity clinics and programs: results and recommendations. Pediatrics 2011; 128(Suppl 2):S59–64.
8. Dykes JC, Kipps AK, Chen A, et al. Parental acquisition of echocardiographic images in pediatric heart transplant patients using a handheld device: a pilot telehealth study. J Am Soc Echocardiogr 2019;32:404–11.
9. Chen AC, Rosenthal DN, Couch SC, et al. Healthy hearts in pediatric heart transplant patients with an exercise and diet intervention via live video conferencing-Design and rationale. Pediatr Transplant 2018;23:e13316.

Building a Viable Telemedicine Presence in Pediatric Rheumatology

Rajdeep Pooni, MD[a],[*],[1], Christy Sandborg, MD[a],[1],
Tzielan Lee, MD[a],[1]

KEYWORDS

- Pediatric rheumatology access • Telemedicine in pediatric rheumatology
- Clinical examination telemedicine

KEY POINTS

- This article describes issues in patient access to pediatric rheumatologic care and the potential use of telemedicine in pediatric rheumatology. It also describes the necessary components of clinical exams in pediatric rheumatology.

In pediatric rheumatology, patient access to certified providers is a troubling issue. The Arthritis Foundation estimates that approximately 300,000 children in the United States have juvenile idiopathic arthritis (JIA), but notes that there are fewer than 400 board-certified and practicing pediatric rheumatologists.[1] There are presently 9 states (including Alaska, Idaho, Montana, New Hampshire, Oklahoma, South Dakota, Wyoming and West Virginia) that are without any full-time pediatric rheumatology providers (**Fig. 1**).[2,3] The American Academy of Pediatrics Division of Workforce and Medical Education Policy notes that most pediatric subspecialists are working in urban areas, at academic centers, with median wait times that may exceed 2 weeks for some specialties.[4] In pediatric rheumatology, this means that patients are traveling an average of 92 km (57 miles)[5] to see their provider, compared with 40 km (25 miles) for patients followed in other pediatric subspecialties, and up to a quarter of adult rheumatologists care for pediatric patients with rheumatologic needs.[6] This finding represents a considerable gap in access because most pediatric rheumatic diseases are chronic cyclic conditions. With respect to patient adoption of telemedicine, another study in pediatric rheumatology reported that, even though 28% of clinic patients traveled greater than 3 hours to see their pediatric rheumatology providers, most (95%) patients reported preference for in-person clinical visits rather than telemedicine visits.

---

[a] Pediatric Rheumatology, Lucile Packard Children's Hospital, Stanford, CA, USA
[1] Present address: 700 Welch Road, Suite 301, Palo Alto, CA 94304.
[*] Corresponding author.
E-mail address: rpooni@stanford.edu

Pediatr Clin N Am 67 (2020) 641–645
https://doi.org/10.1016/j.pcl.2020.04.006   **pediatric.theclinics.com**

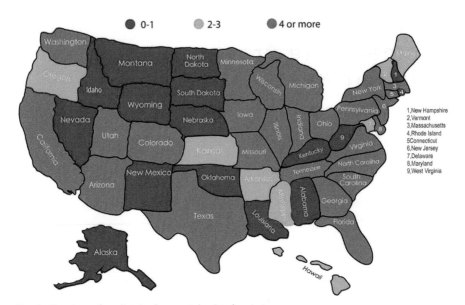

Fig. 1. Number of pediatric rheumatologists by state.

However, patient familiarity with telemedicine as a clinical tool did increase the preference for telemedicine visits.[7] Before telemedicine practices can be adopted as a routine part of pediatric rheumatology care, providers and patients need to clearly understand its strengths and limitations as a tool for health care. For providers, this includes research that results in standardization of telemedicine practices, including (1) specification of patients appropriate for telemedicine follow-up, and (2) clinical guidelines for conducting appropriate and complete video examinations. For patients and their families, this may include education around telemedicine and planning for incorporating telemedicine as part of their routine chronic disease management.

Standardizing telemedicine clinical practice in pediatric rheumatology still needs to be done to ensure appropriate and comprehensive care is given to patients with chronic disease, as well as providing standardized workflows that can support governmental initiatives and policies surrounding telehealth. In order to address the provider-specific issues related to telemedicine, the key issues that have limited its adoption as a part of pediatric chronic disease management have begun to be unpacked.

The pediatric rheumatology group at Stanford Children's has already begun to study this problem and is in the first part of a multiphase pilot study that addresses the clinical gaps involved in pediatric rheumatology provider-patient video visits. Based on expert input, we have identified barriers to adoption of telemedicine that surround the components of the in-person clinic visit experience, including but not limited to (1) the rheumatologic physical examination, (2) the vital signs, (3) modes of communication between provider and patient, (4) the need for immediate laboratory work or imaging, and (5) the need for nursing or social work support. The first phase of the study used expert clinical opinion with modified Delphi methodology[8] to establish what is standard of practice and essential to clinical practice in routine, follow-up, in-person appointments for patients with either JIA or systemic lupus erythematosus (SLE). The reason for selection for patients with these diagnoses is that (1) they are the most commonly treated diagnoses in pediatric rheumatology clinical practice, and (2) they differ in terms of clinical assessment of disease activity. For example, in

SLE, a patient may not have overt clinical symptoms of active disease but may have laboratory features that suggest otherwise, whereas a patient with JIA may have completely normal laboratory tests but a large swollen knee. This process included independent ratings of a 16-item survey on present clinical practices by a panel of 4 attending pediatric rheumatologists at Stanford Children's Health, followed by a face-to-face meeting to reach consensus regarding those survey items that did not reach at least 75% consensus (per item) in the written survey. Each item that had not reached consensus in the initial written survey was reviewed and discussed, and consensus for all survey items was reached in the first round of discussion. As shown in **Box 1**, immediate access to clinic resources such as laboratory, social work, nursing, and imaging is convenient to have but not necessary for most of our follow-up patients with JIA or SLE. Furthermore, the essential examination components that help determine disease activity, disease progression, or medication side

---

Box 1
Necessary clinical components for pediatric rheumatology visits

Essential components for SLE follow-up visit

Vitals: temperature, blood pressure, weight
  Examination:
    Focused ear, nose, and throat examination
    Lung examination
    Cardiac examination
    Abdominal examination
    Skin examination
    MSK/joint examination: general upper extremities and lower extremities
  Laboratory tests:
    Laboratory tests are necessary to determine level of disease activity
    Laboratory tests are not necessary at the time of the clinical visit but are needed for that encounter
  Imaging
    Imaging is not required at time of the visit in greater than 50% of patients with SLE

Essential components for JIA[a] follow-up visit

Vitals: weight
  Examination
    Lung examination
    Cardiac examination
    Abdominal examination
    MSK/joint examination including:
    Temporomandibular joint
      Spine/sacroiliac joints
      Upper extremities
      Lower extremities
      Leg length
      Gait
  Ophthalmologic examination[b]
  Laboratory tests:
    Laboratory tests are not necessary to determine level of disease activity
    Laboratory tests are not necessary at the time of the clinical visit, but may be needed for that encounter (ie, drug toxicity monitoring)
  Imaging
    Imaging is not required at the time of the visit in more than 50% of patients with SLE

Abbreviation: MSK, musculoskeletal. [a] If systemic JIA, need blood pressure, temperature, and weight. [b] For known iritis, need documentation from ophthalmologist within last 3 months.

effects vary depending on the diagnosis and characteristics of the individual patient's disease. For example, a patient with known JIA and uveitis needs regular eye examinations. The slit-lamp examination is critical for monitoring uveitis activity; however, it is within routine practice for rheumatologists to conduct a basic ophthalmologic examination because chronic changes may be visible without slit-lamp. The essential components for a rheumatologic clinical examination are featured in **Box 1**.

The next steps of this study are to use the clinical framework outlined in **Box 1** and develop a checklist, that will be used to directly compare follow-up video visits and follow-up in-person visits in the Stanford Children's pediatric rheumatology clinics. We hypothesize that 75% of the essential clinical standard practice (including examination) will be completed in the telemedicine visits. Ultimately, we will be able to measure these differences and understand the specific limitations of patient-provider video visits, such as effectiveness for urgent problems that come up unexpectedly. Understanding the differences between both types of clinical visits will (1) help determine solutions toward potential examination limitations, (2) provide a framework that can be used to standardize video visits, (3) understand the necessary education for patients around video visits, (4) improve provider clinical support and education regarding telemedicine visits, and (5) further governmental policy or insurance practices regarding telemedicine reimbursement.

If pediatric rheumatologists can better understand what is essential and nonessential in an in-person clinic visit, they can better understand the potential limitations in the use of telemedicine for chronic disease management and work toward solutions that continue to increase access and improve medical decision making in telemedicine.

The study described earlier and preliminary data show the need for additional research in telemedicine in pediatric rheumatology care. Only by understanding how to optimally use technologic tools can clinicians improve the delivery of medical care for patients with chronic disease. Telemedicine in pediatric rheumatology care can serve as a model for other pediatric subspecialties requiring chronic disease management. Studies could be conducted in other subspecialties, because the necessary clinical components for successful follow-up visits may vary widely. Telemedicine has the potential to be a critical component in pediatric chronic care, and it is the responsibility of clinicians to understand how best to use it for their patients.

ACKNOWLEDGMENTS

The authors acknowledge the following groups and individuals for their partnership and research guidance: Pediatric Rheumatology Department, Stanford Children's Health, Health Research and Policy Department, Stanford University. C. Jason Wang MD PhD, Director of Center for Policy, Outcomes and Prevention, Stanford. Lee Sanders MD MPH, Associate Professor of Pediatrics, Lucile Packard Children's Hospital, Stanford.

DISCLOSURE

The authors have nothing to disclose.

REFERENCES

1. Battafarano DF, Ditmyer M, Bolster MB, et al. 2015 American College of Rheumatology Workforce Study: Supply and Demand Projections of Adult Rheumatology Workforce, 2015–2030. Arthritis Care Res 2018. https://doi.org/10.1002/acr.23518.

2. Available at: https://my.rheumatology.org/find-a-rheumatologist. Accessed February 8, 2020.
3. Pediatric Rheumatologists by State - Google Search. Available at: https://www.google.com/search?sxsrf=ACYBGNTIP4J_S2F5Xwu6dRtzTN9NCIF1oQ%A1581483441235&source=hp&ei=sYVDXtL5C8XC-gSa0JyQCw&q=pediatric+rheumatologists+by+state&oq=pediatric+rheumatologists+by+state&gs_l=psy-ab.3..0i22i30.3159.8283..8461...3.0..0.107.2805.34j1. Accessed February 8, 2020.
4. Rimsza ME, Ruch-Ross HS, Clemens CJ, et al. Workforce Trends and Analysis of Selected Pediatric Subspecialties in the United States. Acad Pediatr 2018. https://doi.org/10.1016/j.acap.2018.04.008.
5. Increase Access to Pediatric Rheumatologists. Available at: http://www.arthritis.org/advocate/our-policy-priorities/access-to-care/increase-access-to-pediatric-rheumatologists/. Accessed September 29, 2019.
6. Mayer ML, Mellins ED, Sandborg CI. Access to pediatric rheumatology care in the United States. Arthritis Rheum 2003. https://doi.org/10.1002/art.11462.
7. Bullock DR, Vehe RK, Zhang L, et al. Telemedicine and other care models in pediatric rheumatology: An exploratory study of parents' perceptions of barriers to care and care preferences. Pediatr Rheumatol 2017. https://doi.org/10.1186/s12969-017-0184-y.
8. Ilowite NT, Sandborg CI, Feldman BM, et al. Algorithm development for corticosteroid management in systemic juvenile idiopathic arthritis trial using consensus methodology. Pediatr Rheumatol 2012. https://doi.org/10.1186/1546-0096-10-31.

Telehealth Opportunities and Challenges for Managing Pediatric Obesity

Victor Cueto, MD, MS[a],*, Lee M. Sanders, MD, MPH[b]

KEYWORDS

- Pediatric obesity • Telehealth • mHealth

KEY POINTS

- Telehealth offers an acceptable and feasible approach for the treatment of pediatric obesity.
- Telehealth can address the unmet needs and common challenges of clinical care for pediatric obesity.
- Telehealth for pediatric obesity has the potential to improve access to care, engagement and satisfaction with care.

INTRODUCTION

The treatment and management of pediatric obesity is challenging. The cornerstone of medical treatment for pediatric obesity aims to promote lifestyle modification through the support of behavioral changes involving dietary and physical activity habits.[1–3] The most effective interventions are comprehensive behavioral programs that include multiple components, delivered by a multidisciplinary team, and involve a large amount of contact hours as well as a high frequency of visits between patients, families, and providers.[3] These comprehensive programs require considerable care coordination, and a significant investment of time, transportation, effort, and resources. Unfortunately, this model of care is often inconvenient, burdensome, and inaccessible, particularly for patients and families in underserved or rural communities.[4–7] Furthermore, the number of patients and families who need intensive behavioral therapy exceed the number of appropriately trained primary care providers and tertiary care centers available to offer services.[8,9] Ultimately, access to treatment is limited and programs suffer from poor patient engagement and a high degree of attrition.[10,11] Telehealth holds significant promise for overcoming each of these challenges and has the potential to

[a] Division of General Internal Medicine, Department Internal Medicine, Rutgers New Jersey Medical School, 150 Bergen Street, Room H-251, Newark, NJ 07103, USA; [b] Division of General Pediatrics, Department Pediatrics, Stanford University School of Medicine, 1265 Welch Rd, 240x, Stanford, CA 94305, USA
* Corresponding author.
E-mail address: victor.cueto@rutgers.edu

Pediatr Clin N Am 67 (2020) 647–654
https://doi.org/10.1016/j.pcl.2020.04.007
0031-3955/20/© 2020 Published by Elsevier Inc.

address geographic and logistical barriers, as well as improve access to primary care practices and tertiary care centers.

TELEHEALTH IN PRACTICE OF PEDIATRIC OBESITY

Telehealth is particularly well suited for pediatric obesity because the diagnosis, treatment, and ongoing management of this condition is not usually dependent on a physical examination or physical presence. Telehealth approaches to pediatric obesity are inclusive of a wide range of modalities, including human-to-human interactions via remote visits, interactive human-to-human text messaging, automated and algorithmic messaging independent of human contact, interactive mobile applications (apps), and multiple combinations of these and other emerging technologies.[12–20] Tradition has established the current practice of in-person visits and evaluations, yet there is arguably little in regard to the assessment and ongoing management of pediatric obesity that could not be accomplished using telehealth.

Telehealth Diagnosis and Assessment

Telehealth approaches may enhance the efficiency of obesity diagnosis and assessment. The initial evaluation of obesity is inclusive of a comprehensive history and thorough review of growth and weight trajectory, and an assessment of weight, height, blood pressure, and physical examination by well-trained professionals. Telehealth may be particularly well suited for the collection of important components of the initial evaluation, such as obtaining a family history, current and past medication use, past experience with self-directed or supervised weight management interventions, social history and home environment, sleep history, and an accurate record of usual dietary and physical activity habits.

Ongoing assessment of pediatric obesity through telehealth is made using reliable measurements of height and weight, and blood pressure, collected remotely at settings other than a clinic, such as at home or in a school health office. Bluetooth-enabled devices, such as scales and blood pressure cuffs, may transfer these measurements remotely to the medical record.

Telehealth may also aid the assessment of key physical examination findings pertinent to obesity and related comorbidities, such as acanthosis nigricans, hirsutism, intertrigo, or striae, which could be reliably ascertained through a telehealth format that incorporates synchronous video technology or asynchronous high-definition image technology. However, in-person visits may still be necessary to assess and monitor examination findings, such as lymphedema or joint tenderness, that require touch or advanced examination techniques.

Diagnostic evaluation for rare endogenous or exogenous causes of obesity and laboratory screening for common comorbid conditions, such as dyslipidemia, nonalcoholic fatty liver disease, polycystic ovarian syndrome, and metabolic syndrome, could also be accomplished using telehealth platforms that are integrated with electronic medical records.

Approach to Telehealth Treatment

The aim of medical treatment of pediatric obesity is to promote lifestyle modification and support behavior change. The essential components of effective interventions for pediatric obesity in primary care, specialty, and comprehensive behavioral programs involve providing education and information regarding diet and exercise behavior, while supporting ongoing self-monitoring, goal setting, and problem solving.[1–3] Clinical interventions may be delivered through individual or group sessions involving parents and children, separately or together. The components of the traditional in-person treatment model for pediatric obesity are entirely compatible with a telehealth approach, and may perhaps be more efficiently delivered using telehealth.

Beyond translating existing in-person treatment approaches to telehealth, the incorporation of additional established and emergent technologies into pediatric obesity care may serve to support and augment care. Specifically, the use of wearable devices (eg, smart wristbands, smart watches) and mobile apps (eg, health tracking software) may facilitate self-monitoring and improve personalization of treatment regimens.[12] These mobile technologies may also provide clinicians and patients with more continuous and richer data that can support individual behavior change and feedback, as well as assist clinicians with population health management.

Aside from medical treatment, the use of telehealth for pediatric obesity has also involved using telehealth modalities to support prebariatric and postbariatric surgery activities. Bariatric surgery is recommended and highly efficacious for adolescents and young adults who have not improved with lifestyle modification or suffer from severe obesity and comorbidities.[2,21] Telehealth has shown utility for delivering interventions and supporting the clinical care of patients before and after surgical procedures by facilitating treatment components, such as exercise and preventing regain of weight.[22,23]

Telehealth Treatment Models and Modalities

There have been limited published reports of telehealth modalities for the clinical treatment of pediatric obesity. However, the existing evidence from research studies and clinical practice have shown that a telehealth approach to treatment is feasible, well accepted, and comparable with traditional in-person care.[14–16] Studies and clinical practice models have incorporated multiple telehealth modalities including telephone, text messaging, and live video. These telehealth approaches have been heterogeneous in their involvement of staff, including physicians, specialists, dietitians, and health coaches. Similarly, treatment models have differed in that some have used direct telehealth, where a provider communicates with patients and families, whereas others have used teleconsultation, whereby a specialist supports care and provides consultation.

Studies highlighting different telehealth modalities and telehealth clinical models are presented in **Table 1**. These studies were selectively chosen as examples of the wide heterogeneity of technologies and staffing models used in treating obesity using telehealth. Additionally, these studies also showcase a few important findings and lessons learned in the implementation of telehealth for rural and urban populations, and the role of telehealth for improving access to services. These examples of telehealth implementation in the clinical practice of pediatric obesity underscore the utility of the approach, its potential benefits as compared with traditional care, and the unmet needs that motivate use.

Because of the geographic barriers to care and high prevalence of obesity in rural areas, a considerable proportion of telehealth studies in pediatric obesity have involved rural settings. A randomized controlled study of a rural population by Davis and colleagues[14] is notable for finding outcomes to be comparable between telemedicine visits from psychologists and traditional visits by primary care physicians. Another rural study by Irby and colleagues,[18] which showcases an obesity clinic innovation that adapted an existing tertiary clinical model to a telemedicine format, found that the telemedicine program considerably increased access to care while maintaining comparable engagement and clinical outcomes, as compared with the traditional program. Studies that have examined satisfaction with telehealth for pediatric obesity

Table 1
Selected studies highlighting telehealth modalities and models for pediatric obesity

Modality	Study/Setting	Care Model	Lessons Learned	Author
Tele-visits	RCT, Rural	PCP visits vs psychologist tele-visits	Comparable attrition; Telemedicine encounter similar to face-to-face per psychologists; Comparable outcomes	Davis et al,[14] 2013
Tele-visits	Observational, Rural	Specialist clinic visits vs specialist tele-visits	Increased access; Comparable outcomes; Comparable attrition	Irby et al,[18] 2012
Tele-visits	RCT, crossover, Urban	PCP visits vs PCP visits + specialist tele-visit	Increased access; Time saved for work/school; Preference for tele-visits	Fleischman et al. Fleischman A, Hourigan SE, Lyon HN, et al. Creating an Integrated Care Model for Childhood Obesity: A Randomized Pilot Study Utilizing Telehealth in a Community Primary Care Setting. Clin Obes. 2016;6(6):380-388. doi:10.1111/cob.12166
Tele-visits	Observational Survey, Urban	Specialist clinic vs specialist tele-visits	No difference in satisfaction	Mulgrew et al,[16] 2011
Mobile app, Tele-visits	Observational Retrospective cohort	Health coaches	High level of engagement; Low level of attrition; Change in weight status	Cueto et al,[17] 2019
Tele-visits, Texting	RCT, Urban	PCP + text vs PCP + text + health coach (tele/in-person)	Feasible and well accepted; Comparable outcomes; Greater satisfaction with health coaching	Taveras et al,[15] 2017
Tele-visits, Texting, GIS mapping	RCT, Urban	PCP + text vs. PCP + text + health coach (tele/in-person)	High satisfaction; Parents recommend video tele-visits; Travel cost and time savings; Tele-visits promoted face-face interaction	Bala et al,[13] 2019

Abbreviations: PCP, primary care provider; RCT, randomized controlled trial; GIS (geographic information system); tele, telehealth.

have either found no difference in satisfaction between traditional care and telehealth or improved satisfaction with telehealth.

A recent analysis by Bala and colleagues[13] of secondary data from a randomized controlled trial that used health coaching video visits, found video visits to be well received and accepted by families. The primary reasons reported for satisfaction with health coaching video visits included savings on travel costs and time, and the ability to have a face-to-face interaction. Overall, implementation of different telehealth modalities in clinical practice and clinical research interventions has been reported to be well accepted and satisfying for participants, increase access, save time and cost, and have comparable outcomes to traditional care.

Outside of clinical practice, the broader field of telehealth involving mobile devices and mobile health (mHealth) in pediatric obesity is fairly nascent. The bulk of pediatric studies have used text messaging and mobile apps as adjunctive or supportive elements of multicomponent interventions.[12] In a supportive role, text messaging and mobile devices have been shown to be feasible in aiding self-monitoring and promoting behavior changes related to pediatric obesity. Of note, the evidence for messaging technology, digital health, and mHealth is more robust for adults than pediatrics. Scalable and affordable evidence-based modalities in this field include unidirectional text messaging, bidirectional messaging, artificial intelligence enabled interactions, and fully automated approaches.[24,25] However, there is a lack of evidence for mHealth solutions as stand-alone modalities for treatment in pediatrics.[12] Similarly, research has shown that most mobile apps targeting pediatric obesity are commercially available, but not evidence-based or informed by expert recommendations.[26,27] This is an area of active research with ongoing studies and emerging research.[28–30]

Mobile devices have the potential to integrate multiple telehealth modalities, such as text messaging, telemedicine video visits, and mobile apps. This is evidenced in our study examining a commercial program consisting of multiple components including health coaching through video sessions, text messaging with health coaches, and self-monitoring through a mobile app platform, which found that participants maintained a high level of engagement, with a low degree of attrition, and a change in weight status associated with the number of coaching sessions received.[17] These findings suggest that mHealth solutions that integrate multiple modalities may emerge as an option for stand-alone treatment or a new avenue for providing clinical care for pediatric obesity using telehealth. The utility and role of multimodal mHealth platforms warrants further research.

Research Opportunities

Several ongoing controlled studies are testing the efficacy of telehealth modalities for obesity prevention and treatment.[28–30] Further clinical and population-based research is necessary to assess the utility and effectiveness of emerging telehealth innovation and treatment protocols. Comparative effectiveness studies should examine the relative contribution of different telehealth modalities to improve health outcomes (eg, blood pressure and adiposity) and comorbidities, and promote health behavior change (eg, dietary and physical activity). Potential research questions include the following:

- What is the utility of telehealth by provider type (eg, primary care, health coach, obesity specialist)?
- What is the comparative benefit of synchronous, asynchronous, and combined models of telehealth care?
- What is the relevant impact of different independent and combined telehealth approaches (eg, tele-visits, video coaching, text messaging, or mobile apps)?

Implementation science studies should explore models of telehealth in clinical practice that incorporate evidence-based protocols with different staffing patterns and treatment regimens with varying frequency of visits. Clinical intervention and population level studies should also examine the impact of telehealth on health disparities and underserved groups. A particular hypothesis to be explored is whether telehealth may be especially beneficial for low-income patients and families, for whom time away from work and school devoted to in-person visits may represent a disparate financial burden.

FUTURE OF TELEHEALTH IN PEDIATRIC OBESITY

The incorporation of telehealth in the care of pediatric patients with obesity is ongoing and evolving, with a significant degree of variability in clinical practice. The future of telehealth for pediatric obesity should include primary and tertiary care clinical settings. Health systems and clinicians should continue to explore the utility of telehealth to innovate and support in-person models, and inspire new models of care. The implementation of telehealth as a stand-alone model would take the field in a new direction. The redesign of existing clinical care practices and the creation of new programs must aim to align patient needs with access to care and workforce expertise. Ultimately, the economic viability of telehealth for pediatric obesity depends on the reimbursement of services and the relevant policies of insurers, individual states, and the federal government.[31] This is particularly true for federally qualified health centers, who provide care for the underserved, but are significantly influenced by and dependent on state Medicaid policies for expanding the scope and reach of telehealth services.[31] Telehealth implementation and reimbursement is an active focus of the Centers for Medicare and Medicaid Services, and recent guidance from Medicaid and new policies for Medicare have helped inform clinicians and health systems.[32,33] Presently all 50 state Medicaid programs provide some type of reimbursement for live video services.[34] However, federal statute, Medicaid rules, and state laws allow considerable flexibility regarding which telehealth services individual state Medicaid programs cover. Clinicians who provide pediatric obesity services for Medicaid beneficiaries should advocate for the establishment of a recognized and reimbursable treatment regimen similar to the intensive behavioral therapy program approved for adult Medicare beneficiaries.[35]

SUMMARY

Telehealth is well positioned to address the common challenges of providing high-quality care to children and adolescents with obesity. The potential benefits of telehealth for pediatric obesity are applicable across the full spectrum of care from diagnosis and assessment to ongoing management. Overall, telehealth models of care for pediatric obesity may improve access to care, are feasible and comparable with in-person programs, and are satisfying and engaging for patients and families.

REFERENCES

1. Barlow SE. Expert committee recommendations regarding the prevention, assessment, and treatment of child and adolescent overweight and obesity: summary report. Pediatrics 2007;120(Supplement 4):S164–92.
2. Styne DM, Arslanian SA, Connor EL, et al. Pediatric obesity-assessment, treatment, and prevention: an Endocrine Society clinical practice guideline. J Clin Endocrinol Metab 2017;102(3):709–57.

3. US Preventive Services Task Force, Grossman DC, Bibbins-Domingo K, Curry SJ, et al. Screening for obesity in children and adolescents: US Preventive Services Task Force recommendation statement. JAMA 2017;317(23):2417.

4. Dhaliwal J, Nosworthy NMI, Holt NL, et al. Attrition and the management of pediatric obesity: an integrative review. Child Obes 2014;10(6):461–73.

5. Skelton JA, Beech BM. Attrition in paediatric weight management: a review of the literature and new directions. Obes Rev 2011;12(5):e273–81.

6. Skelton JA, Irby MB, Geiger AM. A systematic review of satisfaction and pediatric obesity treatment: new avenues for addressing attrition. J Healthc Qual 2014; 36(4):5–22.

7. Sallinen Gaffka BJ, Frank M, Hampl S, et al. Parents and pediatric weight management attrition: experiences and recommendations. Child Obes 2013;9(5): 409–17.

8. Findholt NE, Davis MM, Michael YL. Perceived barriers, resources, and training needs of rural primary care providers relevant to the management of childhood obesity. J Rural Health 2013;29(Suppl 1):s17–24.

9. Lenders CM, Manders AJ, Perdomo JE, et al. Addressing pediatric obesity in ambulatory care: where are we and where are we going? Curr Obes Rep 2016; 5(2):214–40.

10. Hampl S, Paves H, Laubscher K, et al. Patient engagement and attrition in pediatric obesity clinics and programs: results and recommendations. Pediatrics 2011;128(Supplement 2):S59–64.

11. Skelton JA, Goff DC, Ip E, et al. Attrition in a multidisciplinary pediatric weight management clinic. Child Obes 2011;7(3):185–93.

12. Turner T, Spruijt-Metz D, Wen CKF, et al. Prevention and treatment of pediatric obesity using mobile and wireless technologies: a systematic review. Pediatr Obes 2015;10(6):403–9.

13. Bala N, Price SN, Horan CM, et al. Use of telehealth to enhance care in a family-centered childhood obesity intervention. Clin Pediatr (Phila) 2019;58(7):789–97.

14. Davis AM, Sampilo M, Gallagher KS, et al. Treating rural pediatric obesity through telemedicine: outcomes from a small randomized controlled trial. J Pediatr Psychol 2013;38(9):932–43.

15. Taveras EM, Marshall R, Sharifi M, et al. Comparative effectiveness of clinical-community childhood obesity interventions: the connect for health randomized controlled trial. JAMA Pediatr 2017;171(8):e171325.

16. Mulgrew KW, Shaikh U, Nettiksimmons J. Comparison of parent satisfaction with care for childhood obesity delivered face-to-face and by telemedicine. Telemed J E Health 2011;17(5):383–7.

17. Cueto V, Wang CJ, Sanders L. Impact of a Mobile App-Based Health Coaching and Behavior Change Program on Participant Engagement and Weight Status of Overweight and Obese Children: Retrospective Cohort Study. JMIR MHealth UHealth 2019;7(11):e14458. https://doi.org/10.2196/14458.

18. Irby MB, Boles KA, Jordan C, et al. TeleFIT: adapting a multidisciplinary, tertiary-care pediatric obesity clinic to rural populations. Telemed J E Health 2012;18(3): 247–9.

19. Coles N, Patel BP, Li P, et al. Breaking barriers: adjunctive use of the Ontario Telemedicine Network (OTN) to reach adolescents with obesity living in remote locations. J Telemed Telecare 2018. https://doi.org/10.1177/1357633X18816254.

20. Smith JD, Berkel C, Jordan N, et al. An individually tailored family-centered intervention for pediatric obesity in primary care: study protocol of a randomized type

II hybrid effectiveness–implementation trial (Raising Healthy Children study). Implement Sci 2018;13. https://doi.org/10.1186/s13012-017-0697-2.

21. Kelly AS, Barlow SE, Rao G, et al. Severe obesity in children and adolescents: identification, associated health risks, and treatment approaches: a scientific statement from the American Heart Association. Circulation 2013;128(15): 1689–712.

22. Baillot A, Boissy P, Tousignant M, et al. Feasibility and effect of in-home physical exercise training delivered via telehealth before bariatric surgery. J Telemed Telecare 2017;23(5):529–35.

23. Bradley LE, Forman EM, Kerrigan SG, et al. Project HELP: a remotely delivered behavioral intervention for weight regain after bariatric surgery. Obes Surg 2017;27(3):586–98.

24. Steinberg DM, Levine EL, Askew S, et al. Daily text messaging for weight control among racial and ethnic minority women: randomized controlled pilot study. J Med Internet Res 2013;15(11):e244.

25. Foley P, Steinberg D, Levine E, et al. Track: a randomized controlled trial of a digital health obesity treatment intervention for medically vulnerable primary care patients. Contemp Clin Trials 2016;48:12–20.

26. Schoeppe S, Alley S, Rebar AL, et al. Apps to improve diet, physical activity and sedentary behaviour in children and adolescents: a review of quality, features and behaviour change techniques. Int J Behav Nutr Phys Act 2017;14. https://doi.org/10.1186/s12966-017-0538-3.

27. Schoffman DE, Turner-McGrievy G, Jones SJ, et al. Mobile apps for pediatric obesity prevention and treatment, healthy eating, and physical activity promotion: just fun and games? Transl Behav Med 2013;3(3):320–5.

28. Healthy weight for teens - full text view - ClinicalTrials.gov. Available at: https://clinicaltrials.gov/ct2/show/NCT03939494. Accessed October 8, 2019.

29. Group telehealth weight management visits for adolescents with obesity - full text view - ClinicalTrials.gov. Available at: https://clinicaltrials.gov/ct2/show/NCT03508622. Accessed October 8, 2019.

30. Greenlight Plus Study: approaches to early childhood obesity prevention - full text view - ClinicalTrials.gov. Available at: https://clinicaltrials.gov/ct2/show/NCT04042467. Accessed October 8, 2019.

31. Uscher-Pines L, Bouskill K, Sousa J, et al. Experiences of Medicaid programs and health centers in implementing telehealth. RAND Corporation; 2019. https://doi.org/10.7249/RR2564.

32. Telemedicine | Medicaid. Available at: https://www.medicaid.gov/medicaid/benefits/telemedicine/index.html. Accessed January 14, 2020.

33. Telehealth Services | Medicare. Available at: https://www.cms.gov/Outreach-and-Education/Medicare-Learning-Network-MLN/MLNProducts/Downloads/TelehealthSrvcsfctsht.pdf. Accessed January 14, 2020.

34. State Telehealth Laws and Reimbursement Policies Report | CCHP Website. Available at: https://www.cchpca.org/telehealth-policy/state-telehealth-laws-and-reimbursement-policies-report. Accessed January 14, 2020.

35. Intensive Behavioral Therapy (IBT) for obesity | Medicare. Available at: https://www.cms.gov/Outreach-and-Education/Medicare-Learning-Network- MLN/MLNMattersArticles/downloads/MM7641.pdf. Accessed January 14, 2020.

Remote Parent Participation in Intensive Care Unit Rounds

Phoebe H. Yager, MD

KEYWORDS

- Telehealth • Videoconferencing • PICU • Pediatrics • Parent

KEY POINTS

- Although most pediatric intensive care units invite parents to participate in daily rounds and despite the high value parents place on engaging with providers, many families face barriers preventing them from being physically present on rounds.
- Telehealth for remote parent participation on daily rounds offers one solution to this problem.
- Although studies have demonstrated the feasibility of videoconferencing with parents on rounds, barriers threaten the implementation and sustainability of such programs.
- Highly reliable, user-friendly telehealth technologies coupled with adequate human resources to address logistical challenges and clinical champions to affect culture change are key.
- Further research is needed to better quantify the impact of such programs on patient and parent outcomes and to convince hospital leadership to invest in telehealth solutions.

PROBLEM TO BE SOLVED BY TELEHEALTH

Parents whose children are admitted to a pediatric intensive care unit (PICU) suffer significant life disruption and anxiety. The incidence of parental post-traumatic stress disorder has been reported to be 21%.[1,2] Obtaining honest, open, timely, and understandable information from providers is important to parents, with more than 90% of parents in one study identifying communication with clinicians as an important coping strategy.[3] As pediatricians have championed the concept of family-centered care, the literature linking family participation on daily PICU rounds with improved parent satisfaction and decreased parent stress is growing.[4–6]

The 2017 Society of Critical Care Medicine guidelines for family-centered care in the neonatal intensive care unit (NICU), PICU, and adult intensive care unit (ICU) recommend "family members of critically ill patients be offered the option of participating

Department of Pediatrics, Massachusetts General Hospital, 175 Cambridge Street, CPZS-5, Boston, MA 02114, USA
E-mail address: pyager@mgh.harvard.edu

Pediatr Clin N Am 67 (2020) 655–659
https://doi.org/10.1016/j.pcl.2020.04.008
pediatric.theclinics.com

in interdisciplinary team rounds to improve satisfaction with communication and increase family engagement.[7]" Despite most PICUs offering this option and despite the high value parents place on engaging with providers, many families face barriers preventing them from participating on daily rounds.[8] These range from work demands or care for other dependents to transportation difficulties because of long distances, high travel costs, or lack of transportation.[9,10] This has led to the call from the Institute of Medicine to develop programs using today's technology to promote patient- and family-centered care and provide emotional support to families.[11] Telehealth for remote parent participation on daily rounds offers one solution to this problem.

CHARACTERISTICS OF DISEASES/CONDITIONS THAT LEND THEMSELVES TO TELEHEALTH

ICUs operate at a fast pace because of higher acuity of illness with a more dynamic clinical course relative to other environments of care. PICUs see a high number of medically complex children whose parents know the details of their care best. These characteristics, coupled with the fact that most PICU patients rely on their parents as medical decision-makers, make a telehealth solution enabling remote parent participation on daily rounds attractive. A multicenter observational study of family participation in rounds in 10 adult ICUs highlighted the benefit of having family members on rounds to (1) help the team learn about the patient; (2) enable families to participate in time-sensitive, shared decision-making; and (3) facilitate informed consent for various treatments.[12] The PICU is also an environment that experiences a disproportionate number of deaths relative to other care environments. Parents who have experienced the death of a child in the ICU identify honest and complete information, ready access to staff, and communication and care coordination during end-of-life care as three top priorities to improve quality of end-of-life care.[13] For parents unable to be at the bedside during rounds, telehealth can bridge the distance between parent and provider, enabling ready access to staff and the chance to actively participate in the plan of care for their child in real time.

One may ask what the visual dimension of a telehealth encounter offers beyond the audio interface of a simple conference call. PICU nurses and physicians have shared that the visual dimension of telehealth encounters enables them to better gauge parent emotions and level of comprehension thereby guiding a more appropriate response.[8] Nurses describe how helpful it is to demonstrate bedside cares parents will be expected to continue following discharge and visualize the patient's home and troubleshoot potential challenges.[8,14] Likewise, parents given the opportunity to see the care team and their child during remote rounds claim this helps confirm the clinical picture described in rounds, provides reassurance regarding their child's care, and has a positive effect on communication with the PICU team.[8] Another study found that children admitted to a hospital ward or PICU who were able to videoconference with family and friends experienced less stress than those who did not participate in the program.[15] However, a small number of parents report feeling overwhelmed with guilt and helplessness when seeing their child on a screen rather than being present at the bedside.[16]

For PICU patients with longer lengths of stay it is not uncommon for one parent to stay at the bedside while another cares for siblings at home. The ability to simultaneously update both parents on daily rounds with the use of telehealth minimizes misunderstandings and takes the burden off the bedside parent to convey second-hand information without the ability to answer follow-up questions.[17] Furthermore, situations where no parent can be at the bedside until after work may result in sequential updates from cross-covering providers and lack of continuity of care. This may adversely impact the development of trusting parent-provider relationships. Parents of premature infants who participated in remote updates for 5 days in a row in one NICU reported a significant improvement in terms of their impressions of information sharing, overall NICU care, relationships with their infant's doctors and nurses, and overall satisfaction with care compared with before the intervention.[17]

DIFFICULTIES IN IMPLEMENTATION AND LESSONS LEARNED

Although several studies have demonstrated the feasibility of various technologies to enable remote video-based parent participation on rounds, several themes have emerged related to difficulties in implementation and sustainability. Firewalls around hospitals and spotty Wi-Fi can hinder reliable connectivity, and some parents and providers may become discouraged and reluctant to participate in future encounters.[18] One group addressed this problem by adding a cellular data program to loaner iPads for parents.[8] Although this may help, it is costly. Technical difficulties originating on the parent-side of an encounter may also be difficult for hospital staff to troubleshoot because of lack of familiarity with end-user devices. Providing families with preconfigured devices may help, although this solution comes with its own challenge of ensuring safe return of loaned devices.[8] Although publicly available applications, such as Facetime and Skype, may be an attractive solution, none offers a HIPPA-compliant platform for videoconferencing. Nonetheless, Epstein and colleagues[17] found that most parents invited to participate in updates using non-HIPAA-compliant platforms were agreeable. Early involvement of one's institutional legal department to guide the consent process is wise. Regardless of the technology used, substantial human resources are needed to launch a telehealth program. Telehealth coordinators can (1) enroll families in the program, (2) train them how to use the program, (3) perform test calls, (4) coordinate a window of time when the parent and team will meet to round, (5) send text reminders to minimize "no shows," and (6) launch video encounters to minimize delays on rounds.[19] This level of support must continue beyond the duration of any study period to ensure sustainability and may be costly.

Beyond these technological and human resource challenges, many researchers have struggled to obtain team buy-in for remote parent participation in daily PICU rounds because of a perceived disruption to workflow and addition of workload.[14,20] Lost connections, frozen screens, and poor audio are inefficient and contribute to provider stress. Coordinating a time to remotely round with some parents removes flexibility in terms of rounding order for the rest of the unit.[14] Clinical champions can ameliorate some of these issues by educating the team about the benefits of telehealth rounding and establishing acceptable workflow changes to accommodate remote parent participation on rounds.

Lastly, some providers have voiced concern that the screen is distracting, pulling the team's focus away from the patient and onto the remote relative.[14] Setting clear expectations with parents in advance of remote rounds just as providers do with parents joining rounds in-person may minimize lengthy discussions best conducted outside of rounds.

POTENTIAL HEALTH CARE COST SAVING AND OPPORTUNITY COST SAVING FOR PARENTS AND CHILDREN

Although no studies have quantified health care cost-savings associated with remote parent participation in ICU rounds, Gray and colleagues[21] found that very low birth weight infants whose parents participated in an Internet-based telemedicine program providing daily written clinical updates, a message center, a see your infant section, and other educational offerings were more likely to be discharged directly home than to require a costly transfer to a level II nursery at another facility. Beyond potential patient-related health care cost savings, there are potential cost savings linked to health services use for parents. In a study by Thompson and colleagues,[22] parents of children with life-threatening illnesses who reported more severe post-traumatic stress symptoms were more likely to seek physical and mental health services. To the extent that remote participation in daily rounds may reduce parental stress through access to honest, open, timely, and understandable information, it is conceivable that this could reduce the costs and consequences of long-term post-traumatic stress symptoms. Lastly, there may be significant personal cost savings for parents who participate in remote rounds to avoid lost wages, threat to job and health insurance security, extra dependent-care costs, and expensive transportation.[23]

NEXT STEPS FOR FUTURE

The future is extremely promising in terms of new technologies to ensure faster, simpler, more reliable telehealth solutions that minimize workflow disruption while maximizing bidirectional communication between on-site providers and parents unable to be at their child's bedside. Such technological advancements coupled with leadership support and team buy-in are key to sustainable programs. Further research is needed to better quantify the impact of such programs on patient and parent outcomes and convince hospital leadership to invest in telehealth solutions.

DISCLOSURE

The author has nothing to disclose.

REFERENCES

1. Balluffi A, Kassam-Adams N, Kazak A, et al. Traumatic stress in parents of children admitted to the pediatric intensive care unit. Pediatr Crit Care Med 2004; 5(6):547–53.

2. Nelson L, Gold J. Posttraumatic stress disorder in children and their parents following admission to the pediatric intensive care unit: a review. Pediatr Crit Care Med 2012;13(3):338–47.

3. Jee RA, Shepherd JR, Boyles CE, et al. Evaluation and comparison of parental needs, stressors, and coping strategies in a pediatric intensive care unit. Pediatr Crit Care Med 2012;13(3):e166–72.

4. Aronson PL, Yau J, Helfaer MA, et al. Impact of family presence during pediatric intensive care unit rounds on the family and medical team. Pediatrics 2009;124: 1119–25.

5. McPherson G, Jefferson R, Kissoon N, et al. Toward the inclusion of parents on pediatric critical care unit rounds. Pediatr Crit Care Med 2011;12:e255–61.

6. Phipps LM, Bartke CN, Spear DA, et al. Assessment of parental presence during bedside pediatric intensive care unit rounds: effect on duration, teaching and privacy. Pediatr Crit Care Med 2007;8:220–4.

7. Davidson JE, Aslakson RA, Long AC, et al. Guidelines for family-centered care in the neonatal, pediatric and adult ICU. Crit Care Med 2017;45(1):103–28.

8. Yager PH, Clark M, Cummings BM, et al. Parent participation in pediatric intensive care unit rounds via telemedicine: feasibility and impact. J Pediatr 2017; 185:181–6.
9. Brantley MD, Lu H, Barfield WD, et al. Mapping US pediatric hospitals and subspecialty critical care for public health preparedness and disaster response, 2008. Disaster Med Public Health Prep 2012;6(2):117–25. ISSN: 1935-7893. Online ISSN: 1938-744X.
10. Stelson EA, Carr BG, Golden KE, et al. Perceptions of family participation in intensive care unit rounds and telemedicine: a qualitative assessment. Am J Crit Care 2016;25:440–8.
11. Institute of Medicine (IOM). Crossing the quality chasm: a new health system for the 21st century. Washington (DC): National Academy Press; 2001.
12. Au S, Roze des Ordons AL, Leigh JP, et al. A multicenter observational study of family participation in ICU rounds. Crit Care Med 2018;46(8):1255–62.
13. Meyer EC, Ritholz MD, Burns JP, et al. Improving the quality of end-of-life care in the pediatric intensive care unit: parents' priorities and recommendations. Pediatrics 2006;117(3):649–57.
14. Ostervang C, Vestergaard LV, Dieperink KB, et al. Patient rounds with video-consulted relatives: qualitive study on possibilities and barriers from the perspective of healthcare providers. J Med Internet Res 2019;21(3):e12584.
15. Yang NH, Dharmar M, Candace HK, et al. Videoconferencing to reduce stress among hospitalized children. Pediatrics 2014;134:e169–75.
16. Epstein EG, Arechiga J, Dancy M, et al. Integrative review of technology to support communication with parents of infants in the NICU. J Obstet Gynecol Neonatal Nurs 2017;46:357–66.
17. Epstein EG, Sherman J, Blackman A, et al. Testing the feasibility of skype and facetime updates with parents in the neonatal intensive care unit. Am J Crit Care 2015;24(4):290–6.
18. Parsapour K, Kon AA, Dharmar M, et al. Connecting hospitalized patients with their families: case series and commentary. Int J Telemed Appl 2011;2011: 804254.
19. Rising KL, Ricco JC, Printz AD, et al. Virtual rounds: observational study of a new service connecting family members remotely to inpatient rounds. Gen Int Med Clin Innov 2016;1(3):44–7.
20. Yager PH, Cummings BM, Whalen MJ, et al. Nighttime telecommunication between remote staff intensivists and bedside personnel in a pediatric intensive care unit: a retrospective study. Crit Care Med 2012;40(9):2700–3.
21. Gray JE, Safran C, Davis RB, et al. Baby CareLink: using the Internet and telemedicine to improve care for high-risk infants. Pediatrics 2000;106(6):1318–24.
22. Thompson EJ, Anderson VA, Hearps SJ, et al. Posttraumatic stress symptom severity and health service utilization in trauma-exposed parents. Health Psychol 2017;36(8):779–86.
23. Clark ME, Cummings BM, Kuhlthau K, et al. Impact of pediatric intensive care unit admission on family financial status and productivity: a pilot study. J Intensive Care Med 2019;34(11–12):973–7.

Implementing Telehealth in Pediatric Type 1 Diabetes Mellitus

Jennifer L. Fogel, PhD[a], Jennifer K. Raymond, MD, MCR[a,b],*

KEYWORDS

- Telehealth • Telemedicine • Type 1 diabetes mellitus • Pediatric endocrinology
- Chronic disease management

KEY POINTS

- Type 1 diabetes mellitus (T1D) is a lifelong disease requiring intensive glucose, insulin, food, activity, and lifestyle monitoring.
- Pediatric endocrinologists are geographically distributed unevenly, with some patients and their families spending extended time traveling to and from appointments on at least a quarterly basis.
- Telehealth technologies engage patients struggling to attend regular medical appointments.
- Telehealth technologies increase T1D patients' adherence to American Diabetes Association care guidelines and improve their quality of life.

Diabetes is and will remain a major health epidemic in the United States, with a projected increase of 54% to more than 54.9 million Americans living with diabetes between 2015 and 2030.[1] With the growing prevalence of diabetes, there is a reciprocal increase in demand for endocrinologists specializing in diabetes care. Although the Endocrine Society projects that there would be no gap in pediatric endocrinologist supply and demand,[2] there is a substantial uneven geographic distribution of pediatric endocrinologists across the United States, with ratios of children with diabetes to pediatric endocrinologists more than double in the Midwest (370:1), South (335:1), and West (367:1) compared with the Northeast (144:1).[3] Additionally, only 64.1% of US children have access to an endocrinologist within 20 miles, with the percentage going up to only 85.5% within 50 miles.[4] With most pediatric endocrinologists who manage diabetes located in large cities and academic centers, some patients in

[a] Division of Endocrinology, Department of Pediatrics, Children's Hospital Los Angeles, 4650 Sunset Boulevard, Los Angeles, CA 90027, USA; [b] Keck School of Medicine of the University of Southern California, 1975 Zonal Avenue, Los Angeles, CA 90089, USA
* Corresponding author. Division of Endocrinology, Department of Pediatrics, Children's Hospital Los Angeles, 4650 Sunset Boulevard, Los Angeles, CA 90027.
E-mail address: jraymond@chla.usc.edu

Pediatr Clin N Am 67 (2020) 661–664
https://doi.org/10.1016/j.pcl.2020.04.009
0031-3955/20/© 2020 Elsevier Inc. All rights reserved.

rural areas spend a significant amount of time traveling to appointments, with parents and patients missing up to a full day of work and school.[5,6] As with most chronic disease care, the American Diabetes Association recommends that children with type 1 diabetes mellitus (T1D) see their provider or other diabetes team members every 3 months, therefore significantly increasing the amount of time lost from work and school for patients and their families. Telehealth can change the current standard of care, allowing for increased access to providers and improved patient health outcomes in a cost-effective way.

Management of T1D lends itself well to telehealth because current technologies enable frequent communication between patients and their providers, and remote data sharing allows for review and adjustments in diabetes regimens. As with most chronic disease management, patients with T1D are required to have frequent appointments with their providers. With most patients with T1D diagnosed around late elementary or middle school age, telehealth technologies can be used to reach patients who are struggling to attend their quarterly medical appointments. As part of diabetes care management, physical examinations and vital signs likely are not critical for every visit; however, the care team can partner with a patient's primary care doctor if an examination or vital signs are needed, or patients can go to a local pharmacy for blood pressure checks. The required medical information—laboratory testing (eg, hemoglobin A_{1c}) and diabetes device data (from glucometers, insulin pumps, and continuous glucose monitors)—can be collected at a local laboratory and downloaded remotely, respectively, and then shared virtually with the provider.[5–7]

With the implementation of technology specializing in shared medical data, the comparison of telehealth versus in-person provider visits is minimal, with the main difference being the ability to perform a physical examination and take vital signs. Although there is minimal access to devices allowing for routine collection of vital signs via a telehealth appointment, providers have the ability to perform limited virtual physical examinations. Virtual physical examinations can include a general description of the patient, evaluation of work of breathing, skin findings, review of shot and pump sites, and so forth. There are certain telehealth tools that exist to allow for full physical examinations (eg, stethoscope and otoscope), but currently these are not options for routine home-based telehealth care. Another difference between in-person and telehealth appointments is the process for scheduling and connecting patients, which varies by platform.[5,7,8] In general, providers send emails or invitations for a visit. Patients then open and download any necessary apps onto computers or mobile devices. Most platforms allow for patients to enter a virtual waiting room prior to seeing the provider and/or can be seen and connected for a visit only when the provider opens the appointment.

There always are difficulties, challenges, and lessons learned when a new system of doing things is implemented, and telehealth is no different. Challenges arise with training patients and providers on how to use telehealth platforms, complete diabetes device downloads, and order and complete laboratory testing prior to provider appointments.[7,8] Therefore, having team members available for practice sessions prior to first appointments and being accessible to support the telehealth connection troubleshooting before and during visits are recommended. Providers have additional challenges in restructuring visits to ensure all required information is collected as well as addressing any anxiety or hesitation that may occur with implementing a new approach to medicine. Clinics will face their own technical, legal, financial, and documentation challenges that necessitate changes to scheduling, planning of laboratory integration prior to visits, online educational and onboarding resources for patients, new electronic medical record notes, and billing processes that can be slow to implement and require support from the entire hospital. Telehealth clinic visits should be completed in telehealth-only clinics and not mixed with in-person patients, because staying on time with telehealth clinics typically is easier than in-person clinics, due to elimination of the time required for rooming patients, no need to wait for vital signs, and no associated delays due to patients seeing multiple staff members. Additional challenges include ensuring that providers, patients, and their families have adequate Internet access and a private space for visits, that patients need to be within a provider's state of medical license at the time of their appointment, and that currently telehealth laws are different from state to state. Patience and appreciation are necessary for everyone involved while learning a new way to do medicine.

The use of telehealth for routine care has been shown to be equal to if not better than, in a variety of measurements, in-person care. Studies focused on patients with T1D demonstrated that telehealth allows for easier and more frequent contact with medical providers, increasing the population's adherence to American Diabetes Association guidelines and improving their retention in care, especially among young adults facing a challenging transitional period in their lives.[5,7,8] Additionally, telehealth appointments resulted in high rates of care satisfaction,[5–8] significant reduction in the amount of time off required from work and school,[7,8] increase in use of diabetes technologies,[6] and an indication of improved quality of life,[9] with no significant changes in cost.[9] Although these previous studies demonstrated these improvements occurred without a change in hemoglobin A_{1c} levels, Crossen and colleagues[8] recently reported an improvement in glycemic control and adherence to recommended outpatient care among high-risk pediatric patients with T1D participating in telehealth care visits.

Telehealth technology has been used and well accepted for its ability to reach patients struggling to attend routine medical care appointments, including pediatric patients with T1D. It is now time to develop manuals of procedures and best practices, train additional providers to slowly expand the use of telehealth, and adapt the model for implementation in low-socioeconomic-status populations as well as in racial/ethnic minority populations. Finally, telehealth should be considered for use with other alternative care models (such as shared medical appointments[10]) and expanded to care for patients with other endocrine disorders and with other chronic diseases currently managed in traditional medical appointments.

DISCLOSURE

Donaghue Foundation, ID# RGA011022.

REFERENCES

1. Rowley WR, Clement B, Arikan Y, et al. Diabetes 2030: insights from yesterday, today, and future trends. Popul Health Manag 2017;20(1):6–12.
2. Vigersky RA, Fish L, Hogan P, et al. The clinical endocrinology workforce: current status and future projections of supply and demand. J Clin Endocrinol Metab 2014;99(9):3112–21.
3. Lee JM, Davis MM, Menon RK, et al. Geographic distribution of childhood diabetes and obesity relative to the supply of pediatric endocrinologists in the United States. J Pediatr 2008;152(3):331–6.
4. Lu H, Holt JB, Cheng YJ, et al. Population-based geographic access to endocrinologists in the United States, 2012. BMC Health Serv Res 2015;15:541.
5. Wood CL, Clements SA, McFann K, et al. Use of telemedicine to improve adherence to american diabetes association standards in pediatric type 1 diabetes. Diabetes Technol Ther 2016;18(1):7–14.

6. Reid MW, Krishnan S, Berget C, et al. CoYoT1 clinic: home telemedicine increases young adult engagement in diabetes care. Diabetes Technol Ther 2018;20(5):370–9.

7. Raymond JK, Berget CL, Driscoll KA, et al. CoYoT1 clinic: innovative telemedicine care model for young adults with type 1 diabetes. Diabetes Technol Ther 2016; 18(6):385–90.

8. Crossen SS, Marcin JP, Qi L, et al. Home visits for children and adolescents with uncontrolled type 1 diabetes. Diabetes Technol Ther 2020;22(1):34–41.

9. Wan W, Nathan AG, Skandari MR, et al. Cost-effectiveness of shared telemedicine appointments in young adults with T1D: CoYoT1 trial. Diabetes Care 2019; 42(8):1589–92.

10. Bakhach M, Reid MW, Pyatak EA, et al. Home telemedicine (CoYoT1 Clinic): a novel approach to improve psychosocial outcomes in young adults with diabetes. Diabetes Educ 2019;45(4):420–30.

Connected Pediatric Primary Care for At-Risk Children

Barry Zuckerman, MD[a],*, Chun Y. Ng, MBA, MPH[b], Jillian Orr Daglilar, EdM[c],
C. Jason Wang, MD, PhD[d]

KEYWORDS

- Connected health • Telehealth • Pediatrics • Mobile health • Mobile app
- Social risk factors • Biological risk factors

KEY POINTS

- Parental guidance is important, especially for children with social and/or medical risks, but existing evidence-based interventions tend to be resource intensive and difficult to scale.
- Benefits from utilizing the Internet and mobile apps to improve parental guidance of at-risk children include accessibility, convenience, and anonymity.
- Patient-generated data from mobile apps may help identify the most beneficial interventions for improving health interventions and facilitating social changes.

INTRODUCTION: CURRENT ISSUES

Pediatric visits for preventive health care are not long enough to provide all the important information parents need. This issue can be seen by browsing through the hundreds of pages of *Bright Futures* guidelines[1], the American Academy of Pediatrics recommendations for what parents need at their children's different ages. These guidelines are acknowledged to be beyond what pediatricians can provide and should be shared with child and family service community agencies, including home visitors, parent groups, dentists, and schools. Even with this caveat, there still is more information than can be provided consistently in a 15-minute to 20-minute well-child visit. Although the negative impact of inadequate time likely is true for all children and parents, children with biological problems (eg, preterm infants) and/or social problems may be more at risk for poor health and/or developmental issues.

There have been remarkable advances in understanding of how mothers' well-being and social relationships can amplify—and how stress can impair—brain development

a Department of Pediatrics, Boston Medical Center, 801 Harrison Avenue, Boston, MA 02118, USA; b New School for Leadership in Healthcare, Koo Foundation Sun Yat-Sen Cancer, No. 125 Lide Road, Beitou District, Taipei, Taiwan; c WGBH Educational Foundation, 703 New Market Place, Columbia, MO 65203, USA; d Department of Pediatrics, Center for Policy, Outcomes, and Prevention, Stanford University School of Medicine, 117 Encina Commons, Stanford, CA 94305, USA
* Corresponding author.
E-mail address: barry.zuckerman@bmc.org

Pediatr Clin N Am 67 (2020) 665–673
https://doi.org/10.1016/j.pcl.2020.04.010
0031-3955/20/© 2020 Published by Elsevier Inc.
pediatric.theclinics.com

and early learning. The American Academy of Pediatrics,[2] Healthy People 2020,[3] and the Institute of Medicine[4] all recommend that pediatricians strengthen parental guidance for improving children's development and early learning through the adoption of positive parenting techniques. These calls to action are based on evidence that (1) strengthening parenting is essential to promoting the health and well-being of the child,[5,6] (2) pediatric primary care provides opportunities to deliver information because of the near universality of young children visits and the value parents place on their child's providers, and (3) pediatric primary care is important, especially to high-risk children who suffer disproportionately from stressors that interfere with health and development.[2,7] Existing parent-focused guidance provided by pediatricians varies in content and quality, and parents report that it is inadequate in meeting their needs.[8–12] Many of the existing evidence-based parenting interventions (eg, home visiting) are resource intensive, leading to challenges in cost and scalability. These services are important, especially in high-risk populations, whether children are at risk for health and/or for learning and behavioral problems.

The goal of this article is to describe digital media linked to pediatric care to deliver prevention efforts related to 2 specific high-risk groups: low-income and premature infants.

CHARACTERISTICS OF PROBLEMS ADDRESSED

In the following 2 examples of mobile app interventions, both interventions go beyond a focus on the infant to address parental needs, because it is well known that the quality of care mothers provide involves more than informational access; it needs to address the mother's well-being. In addition, both efforts include resources to address social determinants of health by providing information about earned income tax credit, free tax preparation services, family planning, and helpful community organizations.

Mobile technology has become omnipresent and is leveraged to have an impact on health behaviors and outcomes. In the United States, cell phone ownership across all major racial, ethnic, and demographic groups is greater than 90%, including 94% for black and 92% for Hispanic populations.[13] A majority of childbearing women use the Internet as a resource for pregnancy and birth information.[14] Reasons mothers utilize the Internet include convenience, anonymity (especially during pregnancy regarding sensitive topics), entertainment, and community searching to share personal stories and connections.[15] Topic-specific chat rooms and personalized mobile strategies show improved clinical outcomes and can further advance research and precision health interventions.[16–26]

In addition, the use of video as part of mobile technology provides a special benefit to mobile technology and has long been recognized as an important tool for patient education, teaching behaviors, and modeling parent-child interactions.[27–30] The use of video may help maximize the fidelity of an intervention (because it requires minimal facilitation) and can reach and engage mothers more easily than 1-on-1 conversations.[31] In the future, virtual reality and augmented reality potentially will elicit even more engagement. The explicit connection to their baby's provider enhances the potential engagement from mothers. Mothers in focus groups have shared that they open and read/watch information only from people they value.

EXAMPLES OF MOBILE APPS

The development of both apps involved a codesign process between mothers of the target group and other stakeholders (based on their relevance to potential solutions), including clinicians, social workers, infant mental health specialists, and community partners. These groups met multiple times to provide feedback at different stages of development.

Small Moments, Big Impact

Small Moments, Big Impact (SMBI) is a digital platform connected to pediatric primary care to help parents promote their empathy (including self-empathy), hope, and self-understanding. These characteristics lead to responsive mother-child interactions, which are known to be associated with children's social and emotional development, resiliency, and early learning. Because stress,[7,32] depression,[33,34] inadequate social support, poor parental reflection,[35] and fixed mindsets[36,37] can undermine empathy and responsive caregiving, the digital platform involves a 2-generation approach to promoting children's development, early learning, and health.

Mothers will receive an episode of SMBI once a week on their smartphone for the first 6 months of their child's life. The cornerstone of the digital platform is brief videos of a diverse group of families from low-income populations filmed in their homes. In some videos, special and small moments of parent-child interactions for different ages are shown. In other videos, parents share stories about their life, including personal stresses, early life traumas, and aspirations. The video content and accompanied text were codesigned with low-income mothers and clinicians.

Sections of each weekly episode include the following: (1) noninteractive reflection questions following each video, (2) age-related infant development, (3) a mood meter for mothers to record their feelings, (4) 3 interactive questions, (5) a brief video of a pediatrician giving information or of a mindfulness teacher demonstrating activities to reduce stress, (6) cartoons (in response to parents telling us humor is important), and (7) a movie maker that allows parents to take up to five 15-second videos every week that then will be compiled into a video compilation and can be saved to document the baby's progress and the mother's reflections. The app can be viewed at home; however, interested providers may use selected content during an office visit to elicit information about mothers' feelings and life circumstances consistent with what is in the app. At this time, the video prototypes have resonated with parents and providers alike, sparking great conversation and reflection.

A randomized controlled trial pilot is being implemented to evaluate the impact. Outcomes include measures of depression, parental reflection, parenting stress, parental empathy, and a 5-minute recorded play session at 6 months that will be coded for parents' sensitivity and responsiveness to their child. Because this digital platform is scalable due to low costs, widespread dissemination is likely to depend on whether mothers and providers like and value it. In addition, given the increasing need to demonstrate quality and value in an Accountable Care Organization, this digital platform allows providers to improve care for an infant's development without necessarily accruing physician time.

Technology to Advance Children's Health Web Portal

Technology to Advance Children's Health (TeACH) is a Web portal developed to improve the follow-up care for infants born prematurely. Fifteen preterm very-low-birthweight caretakers were recruited from Boston Medical Center and equipped with an iPad or netbook and Internet access. Each caretaker was followed for 6 months after hospital discharge. Each caregiver participated in 5, 30-minute to 45-minute interviews at weeks 1, 4, 8, 16, and 24. These in-depth, semistructured, open-ended interviews were scheduled around the time of the infants' regular appointments. Qualitative methods were used to analyze responses to interviews and forum postings. Quantitative methods were used to analyze daily check-in questions, portal usage, and portal interactivity. Analysis of 71 interviews and parent forum postings showed benefits of emotional support and sharing between preterm families. Participant usage data revealed patterns in time of use (more usage in evenings and late nights [**Fig. 1**]), social network patterns (reciprocity in communications among users [**Fig. 2**]), and positive network externalities (more users lead to more activities [**Fig. 3**]). The authors found that a dedicated preterm portal improved access to condition-specific education and social support and provided a private platform for interacting with patient families.

PretermConnect Mobile App

PretermConnect is a mobile app designed at the Stanford University Health Analytics, Behavioral Interventions, and Technology (HABIT) laboratory to provide real-time interactions for parents of premature infants. The app was developed at the request of parents after the evaluation of the TeACH Web portal. The features of PretermConnect include the following: (1) community to connect mothers of preterm infants to tell their birth stories and for support, (2) forum to ask questions, (3) library with curated health and developmental information, (4) dashboards to record health records and trends, (5) private messaging for 1-on-1 interactions, and (6) push notifications for age-appropriate recommended care and updates.

A logic model (driver diagram) was developed to match PretermConnect features to primary drivers that will improve 4 maternal-child health outcomes: increasedinterpregnancy interval (which is highly correlated to recurrent preterm birth), reduced postpartum depressive symptoms, mother-infant bonding, and breast milk feeding (**Fig. 4**).

Implementation and lessons learned: a codesign process with interviews of 30 mothers (ages 22–38) in Stanford, California (n = 15), and in Pittsburgh, Pennsylvania (n = 15), was performed. Mothers recruited from Stanford were interested in entering their data into the authors' platform, connecting with others who have similarly experienced the trauma of preterm birth, and gaining access to the app's resources and community. Many had high levels of information demand and requested more original

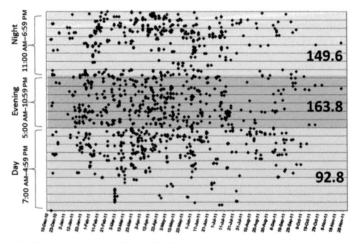

Fig. 1. TeACH Web portal data collected in the time span of a year that shows the distribution of page views during 24-hour periods.

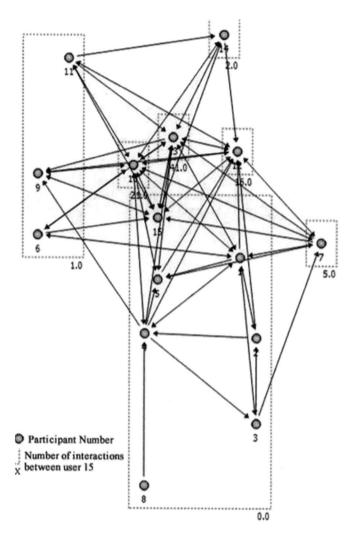

Fig. 2. TeACH Web portal data showing the interaction patterns between participants.

scientific articles. In contrast, mothers from the Pittsburgh area primarily were from low-income families. Most were African Americans from inner-city neighborhoods. Some moms were not as experienced with computers or smartphones (e-literacy) and had difficulties reading articles (health literacy), necessitating lowering the reading level of the articles. Many are using prepaid phones and are at risk of being disconnected. As such, a subsidy of up to $30 per month on a case-by-case basis will be offered for the use of the PretermConnect during the first year of their child's life.

NEXT STEPS FOR THE FUTURE

With patient-generated data from the mobile apps, the authors hope to understand further how engagement and exploration via information and interactions within the apps can lead to social influences, social learning, and social networks that ultimately

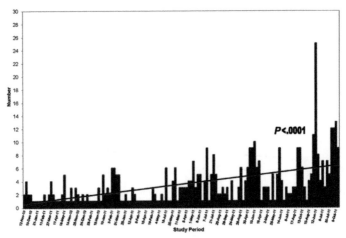

Fig. 3. TeACH Web portal data collected in the timespan of a year showing the number of forum postings on different dates.

can foster trust, social support , and social norms to reduce preterm birth and facilitate better health at the population level.

ACKNOWLEDGMENTS

The authors thank the John Templeton Foundation, the Cabot Family Charitable Trust, the Health Foundation Irving "Harris", and the Janey Fund Charitable Trust for funding and WGBH for partnering to develop Small Moments, Big Impact. This project/publication was made possible through the support of a grant from the John Templeton

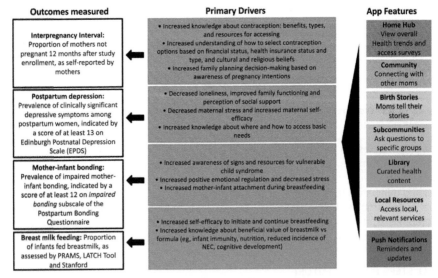

Fig. 4. Driver diagram for PretermConnect that demonstrates how app features could contribute to changes in 4 main measurable outcomes. LATCH, A breastfeeding charting system and documentation tool; NEC, necrotizing enterocolitis; PRAMS, the pregnancy risk assessment monitoring system.

Foundation. The opinions expressed in this publication are those of the author(s) and do not necessarily reflect the views of the John Templeton Foundation. The authors thank the RK Mellon Foundation for funding the PretermConnect project. The authors would like to thank Katherine Edson, Jasmin Ma, and Uma Pulendran for their assistance in preparing and reviewing the article and Shilpa Jani for coordinating the pilot studies for PretermConnect.

DISCLOSURE

The authors have nothing to disclose.

REFERENCES

1. Hagen JF, Shaw JS, Duncan PM. Bright Futures: Guidelines for health supervision in infants, children and adolscents. Elk Grove Village (IL): American Academy of Pediatrics; 2017.

2. Garner AS, Shonkoff JP, Siegel BS, et al. Early childhood adversity, toxic stress, and the role of the pediatrician: translating developmental science into lifelong health. Pediatrics 2012;129(1):e224–31.

3. Healthy People.gov. Healthy People. 2020. Available at: https://www.healthypeople. gov/2020/topics-objectives/topic/early-and-middle-childhood/objectives?topicId=10.

4. National Research Council (US), Institute of Medicine (US), Committee on the Prevention of Mental Disorders and Substance Abuse Among Children, Youth, and Young Adults: Research Advances and Promising Interventions. Preventing mental, emotional, and behavioral disorders among young people: progress and possibilities. Washington, DC: National Academies Press (US); 2009. ISBN-13: 978-0-309-12674-8.

5. Johnson SB, Riley AW, Granger DA, et al. The science of early life toxic stress for pediatric practice and advocacy. Pediatrics 2013;131(2):319–27.

6. Johnston BD, Huebner CE, Tyll LT, et al. Expanding developmental and behavioral services for newborns in primary care: Effects on parental well-being, practice, and satisfaction. Am J Prev Med 2004;26(4):356–66.

7. Shonkoff JP, Garner AS, Siegel BS, et al. The lifelong effects of early childhood adversity and toxic stress. Pediatrics 2012;129(1):e232 LP–246.

8. Coker TR, Windon A, Moreno C, et al. Well-child care clinical practice redesign for young children: a systematic review of strategies and tools. Pediatrics 2013;131(Suppl 1):S5–25.

9. Magar NA, Dabova-Missova S, Gjerdingen DK. Effectiveness of targeted anticipatory guidance during well-child visits: a pilot trial. J Am Board Fam Med 2006;19(5):450 LP–458.

10. Nelson CS, Wissow LS, Cheng TL. Effectiveness of anticipatory guidance: recent developments. Curr Opin Pediatr 2003;15(6). Available at: https://journals.lww. com/co-pediatrics/Fulltext/2003/12000/Effectiveness_of_antici patory_guidance__recent.15.aspx.

11. Norlin C, Crawford MA, Bell CT, et al. Delivery of well-child care: a look inside the door. Acad Pediatr 2011;11(1):18–26.

12. Olson LM, Inkelas M, Halfon N, et al. Overview of the content of health supervision for young children: reports from parents and pediatricians. Pediatrics 2004; 113(Supplement 5):1907–16. Available at: http://pediatrics.aappublications.org/ content/113/Supplement_5/1907.abstract.

13. Pew Research Center. Demographics of mobile device ownership and adoption in the United States. 2018. Available at: http://www.pewinternet.org/fact-sheet/mobile/. Accessed May 14, 2018.

14. Declercq ER, Sakala C, Corry MP, et al. Listening to mothers II: Report of the Second National U.S. Survey of Women's Childbearing Experiences: Conducted January-February 2006 for Childbirth Connection by Harris Interactive(R) in partnership with Lamaze International. J Perinat Educ 2007;16(4):15–7.

15. Romano AM. A changing landscape: implications of pregnant women's internet use for childbirth educators. J Perinat Educ 2007;16(4):18–24.

16. Agarwal S, Labrique A. Newborn health on the Line. JAMA 2014;312(3):229.

17. Schiffman J, Darmstadt GL, Agarwal S, et al. Community-based intervention packages for improving perinatal health in developing countries: a review of the evidence. Semin Perinatol 2010;34(6):462–76.

18. Kumar S, Nilsen WJ, Abernethy A, et al. Mobile health technology evaluation. Am J Prev Med 2013;45(2):228–36.

19. Khoury MJ, Iademarco MF, Riley WT. Precision public health for the era of precision medicine. Am J Prev Med 2016;50(3):398–401.

20. Knight-Agarwal C, Davis DL, Williams L, et al. Development and pilot testing of the Eating4two mobile phone app to monitor gestational weight gain. JMIR Mhealth Uhealth 2015;3(2):e44.

21. Ledford CJW, Canzona MR, Cafferty LA, et al. Mobile application as a prenatal education and engagement tool: A randomized controlled pilot. Patient Educ Couns 2016;99(4):578–82.

22. Evans WD, Bihm JW, Szekely D, et al. Initial outcomes from a 4-week follow-up study of the text4baby program in the military women's population: Randomized controlled trial. J Med Internet Res 2014;16(5):1–12.

23. Whittaker R, Matoff-Stepp S, Meehan J, et al. Text4baby: Development and implementation of a national text messaging health information service. Am J Public Health 2012;102(12):2207–13.

24. Basir M, Ahamed S, Iqbal), et al. The preemie prep for parents (p3) mobile app - a new approach to educating expectant parents who are at risk for preterm delivery. Pediatrics 2018;141(1 MeetingAbstract):17.

25. Ashley EA. The precision medicine initiative. JAMA 2015;313(21):2119.

26. Khoury MJ, Galea S. Will precision medicine improve population health? JAMA 2016;316(13):1357.

27. Gagliano ME. A literature review on the efficacy of video in patient education. J Med Educ 1988;63(10):785–92.

28. Reamer RB, Brady MP, Hawkins J. The effects of video self-modeling on parents' interactions with children with developmental disabilities. Educ Train Ment Retard Dev Disabil 1998;33(2):131–43. Available at: http://www.jstor.org/stable/23879161.

29. Aronson ID, Plass JL, Bania TC. Optimizing educational video through comparative trials in clinical environments. Educ Technol Res Dev 2012;60(3):469–82.

30. Knerr W, Gardner F, Cluver L. Improving positive parenting skills and reducing harsh and abusive parenting in low- and middle-income countries: a systematic review. Prev Sci 2013;14(4):352–63.

31. Fisher PA, Frenkel TI, Noll LK, et al. Promoting healthy child development via a two-generation translational neuroscience framework: the filming interactions to nurture development video coaching program. Child Dev Perspect 2016;10(4):251–6.

32. Gee DG, Casey BJ. The impact of developmental timing for stress and recovery. Neurobiol Stress 2015;1:184–94.
33. Weissman MM, Prusoff BA, Gammon GD, et al. Psychopathology in the children (Ages 6–18) of depressed and normal parents. J Am Acad Child Psychiatry 1984; 23(1):78–84.
34. Hay DF, Pawlby S, Angold A, et al. Pathways to violence in the children of mothers who were depressed postpartum. Dev Psychol 2003;39(6):1083–94.
35. Peter F, Gergely G, Elliot L, et al. Affect regulation, mentalization, and the development of the self. New York: Other Press; 2005.
36. Rowe ML, Leech K. A parent intervention with a growth mindset approach improves children's early gesture and vocabulary de-velopment. Dev Sci 2019;22(4):e12792.
37. Mueller C, Rowe ML, Zuckerman B. Mindset matters for parents and adolescents. JAMA Pediatr 2017;171(5):415–6.

Design, Adoption, Implementation, Scalability, and Sustainability of Telehealth Programs

C. Jason Wang, MD, PhD[a],*, Tiffany T. Liu[b,1], Josip Car, MD, PhD[c,d], Barry Zuckerman, MD[e]

KEYWORDS

- Telehealth • Telemedicine • Design and implementation of telehealth
- Scalability and sustainability • Health care • Health technology

KEY POINTS

- Improving the design and adoption of telehealth may include customization of telehealth services using a human-centered, design thinking process, matching technology to patients' needs, and fixing technological issues such as maintenance of information technology infrastructure, data security and privacy, and interoperability of patient records.
- More robust research on telehealth outcomes that accounts for participant and cost-effectiveness is necessary for its greater adoption.
- The current medical-legal framework for health care delivery is a barrier to scaling telehealth. Policymakers must rethink and address the economic incentives and payment of telehealth services, the medical-legal issues surrounding virtual care, and the effects of increased competition across geographic areas and jurisdictions.

INTRODUCTION

As telehealth programs become prevalent, it is now more urgent and pertinent to ensure its successful integration into the existing health care systems of care. Recently, there has been an increase in consumer technology such as telecommunication tools (eg, Facetime, Skype, WebEx, GoToMeeting, Zoom), as well as a growth

[a] Center for Policy, Outcomes, and Prevention, Stanford University School of Medicine, 117 Encina Commons, Stanford, CA 94305, USA; [b] Center for Policy, Outcomes and Prevention, Stanford University School of Medicine, Stanford, CA, USA; [c] Department of Primary Care and Public Health, Imperial College London, London W6 8RP, UK; [d] Centre for Population Health Sciences, Nanyang Technological University, Clinical Sciences Building, 11 Mandalay Road, Singapore 308232, Singapore; [e] Department of Pediatrics, Boston University School of Medicine, 801 Harrison Ave, Boston, MA 02118, USA
[1] Present address: 117 Encina Commons, Stanford, CA 94305, CA 94305.
* Corresponding author. 117 Encina Commons, Stanford, CA 94305, CA 94305.
E-mail address: cjwang1@stanford.edu

Pediatr Clin N Am 67 (2020) 675–682
https://doi.org/10.1016/j.pcl.2020.04.011
0031-3955/20/© 2020 Elsevier Inc. All rights reserved.

of app-based online consultation platforms (eg, Babylon Health, MDLIVE, LiveHealth, Express Care Virtual). However, matching patients with appropriate technologies and experience remains a significant challenge; patients and providers face additional difficulties navigating virtual care on top of traditional health care delivery. Moreover, telehealth programs need to overcome the lack of traditional face-to-face interaction that allows dialogue to be mapped against facial features and visual cues.[1] Telehealth practitioners should carefully consider the customer experience and their business model; many industries now have both online and off-line presence, such as the retail industry (see the Zappos example in **Box 1**).[2]

In health care, understanding patients' level of interest (or lack thereof) and reasons for using telehealth technologies is only the first step in understanding the full scope and impact of current telehealth programs. Health systems should also consider many more factors when designing and evaluating telehealth care, including human-technology interaction, social factors, technology infrastructure, privacy and security, and organization of health care systems.

DESIGN AND ADOPTION

As technology advances and users continuously adapt to new forms of technology in telehealth, several challenges arise in the design and adoption of telehealth technology. One of the most fundamental aspects of designing telehealth is understanding the patient experience and customizing telehealth to fit user's needs and wants. The first step to holistically capture the patient experience is through the customization and matching of technology to patients. The design thinking process (empathize, define, ideate, prototype, and test) has been widely used as a strategy to assess the needs and wants of users and to rigorously define and test prototypes to develop interventions.[3-10] The most useful telehealth programs benefit greatly from the design thinking process as researchers engage in many iterations of user feedback and customization to tailor programs to fit patients' tastes as closely as possible. At present, this process is often not incorporated into the telemedicine systems; 1 study found that only 61% of information system projects meet customer requirement specifications,[11] and 63% of projects exceed their estimated budgets because of inadequate initial user analysis.[12] Inadequate use of the design thinking may lead to a waste of resources on creating and adopting telemedicine that users do not want or use. However, the design thinking process is often time consuming and expensive, and can be difficult to scale depending on the diversity of patients needed to give appropriate feedback in different practice settings.

One example of successful usage of design thinking in implementing telemedicine is the ongoing telehealth study by the Veterans Health Administration (VHA). The VHA Care Coordination/Home Telehealth network, established in 2003, allows health

---

Box 1
Online Shoe Shopping

One of the fastest-growing industries now is online shoe shopping. Previously, the existence of this industry seemed unimaginable because people assumed that shoe shopping necessitates trying shoes on in person. Zappos, a shoe-selling platform, transformed the customer shopping experience through an innovative new business model of allowing customers to buy multiple shoes online, trying them on at home, and returning ones that they do not want. Its focus on developing customer loyalty and retaining repeat buyers allowed the company to universalize the concept of online shoe shopping.

care providers to customize patient telehealth over multiple years through a combination of remote patient monitoring devices and analysis of ongoing user data and feedback. This comprehensive telehealth program resulted in a 20% reduction in VHA hospital admissions in 2010, and overall patient satisfaction greater than 86% throughout the study.[13] However, this successful implementation required a massive network of providers, robust funding, and years of technology customization. Such individualized customization may be too slow, expensive, and time consuming to scale up. As more telehealth programs are designed and administered, researchers will need to determine ways to select representative patient groups to test their prototypes and efficiently iterate their programs, while balancing available funding for implementation.

Another important issue to consider in telehealth adoption is the need for expansion and improvement in information technology (IT) infrastructure and data security. Rural areas can uniquely benefit from reduced transportation costs from telehealth, but there is often a lack of the broadband capacity to fully implement and scale telehealth in rural regions.[14] In general, expanding telehealth, especially in rural and small practice settings, is hindered by a limited capacity to accommodate bandwidth-heavy telehealth programs. Furthermore, telehealth requires an extensive care team: effective implementation of telehealth often requires receiving and processing data from various devices, which need to be analyzed and translated into clinical information for physicians and other health care providers. Not only are telehealth programs expensive in the installation, operations and maintenance of technological systems also require the hiring and training of key personnel to navigate telehealth technology and to continuously maintain and update IT systems to ensure compliance. Because medical data must be kept private and secure, technology for telehealth often prioritizes defense against security breaches. Telecommunications contain many nodes during storage and transmission, including the device, Wi-Fi routers, Internet service providers, carriers' cellular towers, and cloud storage farms. Each of these nodes contains hardware and software vulnerable to hacking attacks or leaks; therefore, ensuring data security during storage and transit requires stringent privacy policy and security protocols and personnel vigilance.

In addition to complying with the technical requirements, researchers must also account for how technology alters the nature of the patient-doctor relationship. Telehealth practitioners may need to determine an appropriate so-called Web-side manner to account for the loss of a traditional in-person patient-doctor connection. As virtual care becomes more common, care providers must find strategies to make the patients feel comfortable, heard, and understood; to convey empathy and compassion virtually; and to pick up body language or emotional cues from the patients through a screen.[15,16]

OUTCOMES OF TELEHEALTH: EFFECTIVENESS, COST-EFFECTIVENESS, AND PARTICIPANT BIAS

As telehealth solutions are poised to become substitutes for traditional health care services in many clinical arenas, there is a lack of conclusive evidence on the outcomes of telehealth implementation.[17] In a study by the Deloitte Center for Health Solutions, 53% of respondents who have used virtual care visits said that they did not believe the provider they met was as competent or professional as a doctor in an in-person visit. Only a third of respondents said they thought that they had received all the necessary medical information during their virtual care visit.[18] Quality indicators for telehealth care should ideally be developed with input from experts in various specialties of clinical care, quality of care, information technology, and patient representatives. Moreover, gaps in knowledge on telehealth outcomes should include the impact of telemedicine on different patient groups, and over a longer-term period. At present, many telehealth studies have evaluation periods between 6 and 12 months, which might be too short to truly assess the effectiveness of telehealth.[19]

Because of the relative novelty of telehealth, there are few robust studies on the cost-effectiveness of telehealth compared with traditional health care.[19] One study from The UK Whole System Demonstrator project revealed that, after a 12-month implementation of telehealth, there was a reduction in mortality and hospital admissions, but telemedicine was not cost-effective because it served as an add-on to traditional treatments.[20,21] This study challenges the validity of what people regard as a core benefit of telehealth: its ability to replace traditional health care at a much lower cost. Similar to other newly introduced technologies, telehealth programs must establish appropriateness criteria for use to guard against provider or patient overuse and prevent provider-driven demand or moral hazard from patients that leads to increase in health care costs.

In addition, current telehealth research must overcome research sample bias that does not involve a representative, objective pool of participants. For example, people who join telehealth studies tend to already have a positive view of telemedicine. Those who decline to participate worry about health interference, independence, and privacy,[22] all of which are salient barriers to telehealth implementation. Going forward, randomized controlled trials of telehealth in primary care settings, specialty services, and by medical conditions may be necessary to advance the understanding of telehealth.

TRAINING, SCALABILITY, SUSTAINABILITY, AND INTEGRATION
Business Model

There is limited research into a scalable business model for telehealth, and care providers struggle to develop an economically sustainable reimbursement system for telehealth. At present, most states stipulate private insurers to pay for telehealth, but states vary in their requirements of how much those parties ought to pay. For example, some states require insurers to pay for any and all telehealth services, whereas others, such as New Jersey, only require insurers to pay for telehealth programs if they cost less than comparable in-person services.[23] In addition, reimbursements by health insurance programs such as Medicare are not consistent across various types of telemedicine services, and reimbursement policies have not been standardized among various private payers. Furthermore, payers such as Medicare do not recognize the home as a reimbursable originating site of care,[24] except for remote physiologic monitoring.[25] Medicare reimbursement is mostly limited to specific institutions, nonmetropolitan areas, and places with certain current procedural terminology codes.[26]

However, in places with capitated reimbursement, such as the US Veterans Affairs, telehealth programs such as home-based chronic disease management and remote patient monitoring have flourished. Using data from 17,025 patient participants, researchers found a 19% reduction in hospital admissions and a 25% reduction in length of hospital stay through telehealth solutions.[27] It is possible that, in order to overcome barriers to scaling telehealth, new payment and reimbursement systems should be established to align incentives between patients, providers, insurance companies, and other third-parties.

Licensure and Medical-Legal Issues

Another issue hampering wide scalability of telehealth is the licensure and cross-jurisdictional regulations of medical practice. In the United States, most doctors are licensed to practice in their own states,[28] but telehealth can transcend state borders. For certain specialty services with physician shortages, patients cannot reap the benefits of telehealth until health care providers are allowed to offer services to patients outside of their home states, and, in some cases, outside of the country. Regulators should rethink ways to assess eligibility and licensure for telehealth when traditional licensing rules are obsolete in the advent of new technology. They shall also evaluate litigations and other challenges that arise from the medical-legal issues of virtually seeing patients across state borders.

Integrating with Traditional Health Care Services

The emergence of telehealth in the retail space is also worth mentioning, especially with regard to competition within the health care landscape. For example, CVS Health's launch of the MinuteCinic in 2006[29] and Walgreen's 2018 launch of digital health platform Find Care Now signal the expansion of the retail health care market and a shift away from traditional hospital health care.[30] Smaller health care providers may innovate in telehealth to compete with larger health care systems because the value of physical space and infrastructure has depreciated. The inclusion of retail telehealth providers from virtually any geographic location may result in greater competition and erosion of patient loyalty,[31] destabilizing the existing health care system. With the increase in retail telehealth comes new questions about defining ownership of patient-provided data. Many companies may become covered entities under the Health Insurance Portability and Accountability Act (HIPAA), because they now see patients through telemedicine. The lack of clarity regarding the conditions under which personal data become protected health information and the potential legal obligations under existing policies such as HIPAA can impede scalability and sustainability of these platforms if left unaddressed.

Furthermore, integration of telehealth into traditional health care may require challenging adjustments in the current delivery of care. New interorganizational approaches and changes to current health care systems need to be developed because the feasibility and adoption of telehealth services depend on their integration into current organizational practices and workflows,[32] as well as their compatibility with vastly diverse patient populations, physician preferences, and hospital settings.[33,34] One framework to consider is the eHealth-enhanced chronic care model. In this model, physicians involve nurses, pharmacists, or dietitians in coaching the patient through telehealth in between physical hospital visits.[35] This approach combining telehealth with in-person health care can complicate health care delivery, because they require new systems and curriculum for training and management that do not currently exist. Specifically, the lack of proper training and education for medical staff and lack of management support in telehealth impedes implementation of services that incorporate telemedicine into the current health care delivery system.[15,34,36,37] Thus, optimizing care for patients that includes telehealth without detracting from the existing benefits of in-person hospital visits will become an important consideration in the successful scaling of telehealth.

Another barrier to integrating telehealth is the interoperability of patient data; namely, the ability to access, use, and change data across various platforms.[38] The lack of interoperability standards for patient records thereby is an important issue to consider in the integration of telemedicine into health care.[39,40] As people use more diversified telehealth resources instead of 1 central health provider's services, communication and standardization of data across different platforms, service providers, and payer organizations are necessary to protect the integrity of patient data. In a similar vein, the universality of technology invokes the issue of reliability and accuracy, especially for important medical or health information. For example, anyone can make a health app or educational resource that qualifies as telemedicine, but there is currently no system in place to ensure that experts regularly check and verify medically important information. These emergent concerns will define the responsibility and liability of stakeholders, including but not limited to patient users, doctors and nurses, insurance companies, hospitals, and the government regulators.

SUMMARY

Telehealth is a growing health care service with various barriers to successful widespread implementation. To adopt new technologies such as telemedicine, stakeholders often expect strong evidence of potential benefits, which requires longitudinal, comprehensive research. Lack of definitive data on the medical benefits, cost-effectiveness, and cost benefits of telemedicine has been both an economic and social challenge to adoption of telehealth. Improving technological issues such as technology customization and expansion of broadband infrastructure, as well as the reevaluation of the legal processes for handling malpractice claims, privacy and security issues, and data breaches, may be necessary for full adoption of telehealth.

DISCLOSURE

The authors have nothing to disclose.

REFERENCES

1. Rothwell E, Ellington L, Planalp S, Crouch B. Exploring challenges to telehealth communication by specialists in poison information. Qual Health Res 2012; 22(1):67–75.
2. Goldstein S. How Tony Hsieh Transformed Zappos With These 5 Core Values. Inc Mag 2017.
3. Roberts JP, Fisher TR, Trowbridge MJ, Bent C. A design thinking framework for healthcare management and innovation. Healthc (Amst) 2016;4(1):11–4.
4. Eckman M, Gorski I, Mehta K. Leveraging design thinking to build sustainable mobile health systems. J Med Eng Technol 2016;40(7–8):422–30.
5. Beaird G, Geist M, Lewis EJ. Design thinking: Opportunities for application in nursing education. Nurse Educ Today 2018;64:115–8.
6. Velu AV, van Beukering MD, Schaafsma FG, et al. Barriers and facilitators for the use of a medical mobile app to prevent work-related risks in pregnancy: a qualitative analysis. JMIR Res Protoc 2017;6(8):e163.
7. Gorski I, Bram JT, Sutermaster S, Eckman M, Mehta K. Value propositions of mHealth projects. J Med Eng Technol 2016;40(7–8):400–21.
8. Basir M, Ahamed S, Iqbal), Jones C, et al. The preemie prep for parents (p3) mobile app - a new approach to educating expectant parents who are at risk for preterm delivery. Pediatrics 2018;141(1 MeetingAbstract):17.
9. Knight-Agarwal C, Davis DL, Williams L, Davey R, Cox R, Clarke A. Development and pilot testing of the eating4two mobile phone app to monitor gestational weight gain. JMIR mHealth uHealth 2015;3(2):e44.

10. Ledford CJW, Canzona MR, Cafferty LA, Hodge JA. Mobile application as a pre-natal education and engagement tool: A randomized controlled pilot. Patient Educ Couns 2016;99(4):578–82.
11. Williams D, Williams D, Kennedy M. Towards a model of decision-making for systems requirements engineering process management. Available at: http://citeseerx.ist.psu.edu/viewdoc/summary?doi=10.1.1.106.5868. Accessed September 23, 2019.
12. Wallach D, Scholz SC. User-centered design: why and how to put users first in software development. In: Maedche A, Botzenhardt A, Neer L, editors. Software usability in small and medium sized enterprises in Germany: an empirical study. Germany: Springer; 2012. p. 11–38. https://doi.org/10.1007/978-3-642-31371-4_2.
13. Broderick A, Codirector MBA. Case studies in telehealth adoption: the Veterans Health Administration: taking home telehealth services to scale nationally. The Commonwealth Fund 2013;4(1657).
14. Schadelbauer R. Anticipating economic returns of rural telehealth. 2017. Available at: www.ntca.org. Accessed February 10, 2020.
15. van Galen LS, Wang CJ, Nanayakkara PWB, Paranjape K, Kramer MHH, Car J. Telehealth requires expansion of physicians' communication competencies training. Med Teach 2019;41(6):714–5.
16. Heath S. Patients interested in telehealth tech, but improvements are key. Patient Engagement Hit. 2018. Available at: https://patientengagementhit.com/news/patients-interested-in-telehealth-tech-but-improvements-are-key. Accessed February 10, 2020.
17. Currell R, Urquhart C, Wainwright P, Lewis R. Telemedicine versus face to face patient care: effects on professional practice and health care outcomes. Cochrane Database Syst Rev 2000;(2):CD002098.
18. Abrams K, Korba C. Consumers are on board with virtual health options: Can the health care system deliver? Deloitte Insights. 2018. Available at: https://www2.deloitte.com/content/dam/insights/us/articles/4631_Virtual-consumer-survey/DI_Virtual-consumer-survey.pdf. Accessed February 10, 2020.
19. Wootton R. Twenty years of telemedicine in chronic disease management–an evidence synthesis. J Telemed Telecare 2012;18(4):211–20.
20. Dinesen B, Nonnecke B, Lindeman D, et al. Personalized telehealth in the future: A global research agenda. J Med Internet Res 2016;18(3). https://doi.org/10.2196/jmir.5257.
21. Car J, Huckvale K, Hermens H. Telehealth for long term conditions: Latest evidence doesn't warrant full scale roll-out but more careful exploration. BMJ 2012;344(7865). https://doi.org/10.1136/bmj.e4201.
22. Sanders C, Rogers A, Bowen R, et al. Exploring barriers to participation and adoption of telehealth and telecare within the Whole System Demonstrator trial: A qualitative study. BMC Health Serv Res 2012;12(1). https://doi.org/10.1186/1472-6963-12-220.
23. Fanburg JD, Walzman JJ. Telehealth and the law: the challenge of reimbursement. Medical Economics 2018;95(20). Available at: https://www.medicaleconomics.com/article/telehealth-and-law-challenge-reimbursement. Accessed February 10, 2020.
24. Org M, Lazur B, Bennett A, King V. Milbank Memorial Fund • Www the Evolving policy Landscape of telehealth services delivered in the home and other Nonclinical settings issue Brief. 2019. Available at: www.milbank.org.
25. Centers for Medicare & Medicaid Services. Document 2019-24086. Office of the Federal Register 2019. Available at: https://www.federalregister.gov/documents/

2019/11/15/2019-24086/medicare-program-cy-2020-revisions-to-payment-policies-under-the-physician-fee-schedule-and-other. Accessed February 10, 2020.

26. Institute of Medicine. Challenges in telehealth. The Role of Telehealth in an Evolving Health Care Environment: Workshop Summary. Washington, DC: The National Academies Press; 2012. p. 17–30.

27. Bartolini E, McNeill N. Getting to value: eleven chronic disease technologies to watch. 2012. Available at: www.nehi.net.

28. Balestra M. Telehealth and legal implications for nurse practitioners. The Journal for Nurse Practitioners 2017;14(1):33–9.

29. Dalen JE. Retail clinics: a shift from episodic acute care to partners in coordinated care. Am J Med 2016;129(2):134–6.

30. Graham J. Walgreens introduces new digital marketplace featuring 17 leading health care providers. Walgreens; 2018. Available at: https://news.walgreens.com/press-releases/general-news/walgreens-introduces-new-digital-marketplace-featuring-17-leading-health-care-providers.htm. Accessed February 10, 2020.

31. Smith A. How telemedicine technology is changing the competitive landscape. Chiron Health. 2016. Available at: https://chironhealth.com/blog/how-telemedicine-technology-is-changing-the-competitive-landscape/2019. Accessed February 10, 2020.

32. King G, Richards H, Godden D. Adoption of telemedicine in Scottish remote and rural general practices: a qualitative study. J Telemed Telecare 2007;13(8):382–6.

33. Vuononvirta T, Timonen M, Keinänen-Kiukaanniemi S, et al. The compatibility of telehealth with health-care delivery. J Telemed Telecare 2011;17(4):190–4.

34. Al-Qirim N. Championing telemedicine adoption and utilization in healthcare organizations in New Zealand. Int J Med Inform 2007;76(1):42–54.

35. Cueto V, Wang C, Sanders L. Impact of a mobile application-based health coaching and behavior change program on participant engagement and weight status of overweight & obese children: a retrospective cohort study. JMIR mHealth uHealth 2019;7(11):e14458.

36. Lewis ER, Thomas CA, Wilson ML, Mbarika VWA. Telemedicine in acute-phase injury management: A review of practice and advancements. Telemed J E Health 2012;18(6):434–45.

37. Stronge AJ, Rogers WA, Fisk AD. Human factors considerations in implementing telemedicine systems to accommodate older adults. J Telemed Telecare 2007; 13(1):1–3.

38. What is Interoperability in Healthcare? Healthcare Information and Management Systems Society. Available at: https://www.himss.org/what-interoperability. Accessed February 10, 2020.

39. Porter ME, Teisberg EO. Redefining health care: creating value-based competition on results. Boston: Harvard Business Review Press; 2006.

40. Ackerman MJ, Filart R, Burgess LP, Lee I, Poropatich RK. Developing next-generation telehealth tools and technologies: patients, systems, and data perspectives. Telemed J E Health 2010;16(1):93–5. https://doi.org/10.1089/tmj.2009.0153.

Achieving a Quintuple Aim for Telehealth in Pediatrics

Eli M. Cahan, BBA[a,b,]*, Vandna Mittal, MPH[c], Nirav R. Shah, MD, MPH[a],
Sonoo Thadaney-Israni, MBA[d]

KEYWORDS

- Pediatrics • Telehealth • Telemedicine • eHealth • mHealth • Bioethics • Equity

KEY POINTS

- Numerous models of telehealth have been proposed and developed in recent years to combat the increasing prevalence of pediatric complex chronic disease.
- Although these models have shown improvements in care quality, cost, and access, disparities in effectiveness have been noted that negatively affect vulnerable populations.
- Disparities related to telehealth's burden on the workforce serving children and its repercussions on social outcomes have also been noted, so opportunities exist to design a more equitable care delivery paradigm.
- Considerations including judiciousness, acceptability, design, interoperability, effectiveness, dissemination, cost-effectiveness, adaptability, monetizability, and security can help ensure equity amid the further implementation of telehealth serving pediatric populations.

Pediatric practice increasingly involves care for children with complex chronic diseases. Telehealth offers a delivery method via which providers and health care systems can provide direct care, ensure care continuity, coordinate indirect care, and enable other nonmedical services affecting health for children with medical complexity.

However, the fact that telehealth can achieve these positive outcomes does not mean it will do so equitably, especially as it relates to serving vulnerable populations. Without awareness of the potential unintended repercussions on vulnerable populations, and intentionally designing best practices for development, testing, and implementation of telehealth programs, these novel technologies can exacerbate, rather than improve, existing disparities.

[a] Clinical Excellence Research Center, Stanford School of Medicine, Stanford, CA 94305, USA; [b] NYU School of Medicine, New York, NY 10010, USA; [c] Stanford Children's Health, Stanford, CA 94305, USA; [d] Department of Medicine, Stanford School of Medicine, Stanford, CA 94305, USA
* Corresponding author. 366 Galvez Street, Room #322, Stanford, CA 94305.
E-mail address: emcahan@stanford.edu
Twitter: @emcahan (E.M.C.)

Pediatr Clin N Am 67 (2020) 683–705
https://doi.org/10.1016/j.pcl.2020.04.015
0031-3955/20/© 2020 Elsevier Inc. All rights reserved.

pediatric.theclinics.com

This article first describes in brief secular trends related to pediatric chronic disease in the United States. Next, it reviews the evidence available to date supporting the potential of telehealth to address these trends. This article adopts the lens of the Institute for Healthcare Improvement (IHI)'s Triple Aim for health care systems: improvement of outcomes, expansion of access to health care, and reduction in cost.[1] It supplements these principles with 2 others to propose a quintuple aim essential for the effective mass rollout of telehealth: support of the health care workforce, and ensuring equity of the technologies across populations[2] (**Fig. 1**). In addition, harnessing telehealth's opportunity to reduce inequality, it defines a series of core considerations for designing and implementing these technologies to promote optimal care of children in the future.

PATTERNS IN THE PREVALENCE OF, CARE FOR, AND COST OF PEDIATRIC CHRONIC DISEASE
Prevalence

In recent years, chronic diseases have increased as a leading cause of morbidity and mortality in America's children. Some 32 million children, 43% of the total in the United States, have been assessed with at least 1 of 20 leading chronic health conditions.[3] When premorbid conditions such as being overweight, obesity, and early developmental delay are included, more than half of American children (54% of the total) are implicated.[3] Of this chronic disease cohort, more than 14 million (19% of the total population) children have conditions resulting in special health care needs, approximately 1.2 million more than in 2003.[3] Although the prevalence of complex chronic disease has increased overall, the burden disproportionately affects vulnerable populations.[3]

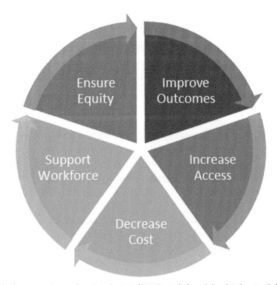

Fig. 1. Framework for a quintuple aim in pediatric telehealth. (*Adapted from* Matheny M, Thadaney-Israni S, Whicher D, Ahmed M. Artificial intelligence in health care: hope not hype, promise not peril. In: Matheny M, Thadaney-Israni S, Whicher D, Ahmed M, editors. AI in healthcare: the hope, the hype, the promise, the peril. Washington, DC: National Academy of Medicine; November 2019 (in press); p. 219. Available at: https://nam.edu/wp-content/uploads/2019/12/AI-in-Health-Care-PREPUB-FINAL.pdf; with permission.)

Disparities in Care Received

However, these same groups face disparities in the care they receive. Nearly two-thirds of publicly insured children with chronic diseases did not receive minimum threshold quality care criteria, a rate 22% higher than privately insured patients.[3,4] Despite the move toward, and American Academy of Pediatrics recommendation for, family-centered care (FCC) in pediatrics, 43% of publicly insured patients did not receive FCC (24% fewer than privately insured).[3,4]

These patterns are also prominent in the children with special health care needs (CSHCN) cohorts who are at increased risk should their care deviate from best practices, because one-third of patients in these groups (regardless of insurance status) fail to receive FCC.[3]

Beyond insurance status alone, racial disparities in CSHCN care quality also have been noted: Latino and African American patients are 47% and 40% less likely to receive FCC, respectively.[5] Similar disparities exist by ethnicity and language, because non–English primary speakers are 52% less likely to receive FCC (even after adjustment for child health, SES, geography, and health care use).[5]

Disparities in Access

Such patterns may arise in part from barriers to access to health care services. Such access deficiencies are not limited to pediatric populations alone: 77 million Americans live in nearly 8000 distinct health professional shortage areas throughout the United States.[6] This figure is 30% higher than it was in 2015.[6]

Previous needs assessments of CSHCNs before the introduction of telehealth found that, in rural regions, 86% and 96% of parents/guardians of CSHCNs had to travel greater than 1 hour and were forced to miss work for appointments, respectively.[7] As a result, nearly one-quarter of American children report difficulty accessing subspecialty care.[3] For 7 of 16 pediatric subspecialties, half of American hospitals have no specialists within their regions.[8] Across subspecialties, the distance to the nearest practitioner is as far as 125 km (78 miles),[8] and families in the lowest wealth percentiles face journeys up to 13 miles longer to receive specialty care.[9]

Overall, 1 in 4 children still has 1 unmet care need, and 1 in 8 has multiple.[10] As a result, families commonly resort to emergency department services, which may or may not fulfill their needs depending on local capabilities.[7]

Cost

Such trends in chronic disease, and the suboptimal care treating it, have produced exceptionally high costs to these families. Although CSHCNs comprise 0.67% of the pediatric population, care for these individuals consumes nearly one-third of the systemic spend; costing 2.5-fold to 20-fold that of the average pediatric patient,[11,12] and accounting for up to 40% of hospitalizations annually.[13]

In addition to direct medical costs, families of healthy children and CSHCNs alike bear substantial indirect costs related to the subclinical aspects of care essential to fulfill the needs of their children (such as routine maintenance, transportation, and care coordination). Studies have found that nondirect medical costs are equivalent to medical costs in healthy children,[14] and, in CSHCNs, up to 90% of care costs for certain cohorts are not direct medical expenditures.[15] These sorts of services are often not covered by insurance programs and accumulate substantial financial burdens on families of children with CSHCNs (one-third to one-half of all costs may be out-of-pocket) and, when lost wages are accounted for, consume some 38% of gross annual family income in certain populations.[15]

THE THEORETIC POTENTIAL OF TELEHEALTH IN PEDIATRICS

Telehealth technologies (including mobile video conferencing, store-and-forward referral systems, mobile applications, and wearable devices) have been identified as a means to address these issues.[16,17] These technologies can improve continuity of primary care, augment access to specialty and ancillary care, and reduce direct and nondirect medical costs.

Mechanistically, this occurs whereby these technologies (1) constitute a digital toolbox of diagnostic and therapeutic instruments for providers and (2) formalize the "curbside consult" between providers across the spectrum of care to (3) form an integrated, virtual, patient-centered medical home.[18,19] Positive uptake of these technologies has been noted in providers, patients, and caregivers/families alike[20–23] (**Table 1**).

THE IMPACTS OF TELEHEALTH ON THE TRIPLE AIM FOR PEDIATRICS

However, telehealth is not necessarily a panacea because of its novelty, sophistication, and good intentions. Presciently, Veinot and colleagues[24] commented that:

> [Telehealth] interventions are designed … to improve the quality and safety of healthcare … Because we have such benevolent goals, we often think the worst thing that could happen is for our efforts to have no effect. However, there is a real and more pernicious possibility: that our technological interventions do work, but they work better for those who are already better off. When this happens, our work actually **increases** [author's emphasis] inequality. This phenomenon, unfortunately well established in public health, is known as 'intervention-generated inequality.'

As such, when evaluating the ripples of introducing telehealth to the pediatric health care system, stakeholders must appraise the potential for these intervention-generated inequalities (IGIs) in vulnerable populations alongside the positive implications of these technologies in mainstream populations. In keeping with the IHI's Triple Aim, the positive and negative influences can be considered on the axes of care quality, cost, and access.

Care Quality

The positive impact of telehealth on health care outcomes has been well documented. In a series by Médecins Sans Frontières (MSF), telehealth showed utility to both patients and providers. For patients directly engaging in telehealth consultations, more than two-thirds of recommendations were deemed useful to self-care.[25] Meanwhile, for providers, more than three-quarters of recommendations made from consulted peers were considered useful: in 64% of referred pediatrics cases, a significant change was made to initial management and, in 25%, a life-threatening condition was recognized that was previously missed.[25,26]

Related to acute conditions, in studies conducted at pediatric intensive care units associated with University of California, Davis, a 19% reduction was noted in observed to expected mortality after risk adjustment following the implementation of telehealth for acute-care consultation.[27] MSF acute-care cohorts observed a 30% reduction in adverse events following introduction of telehealth resources, with a number needed to treat of 45.[26]

Related to chronic conditions, telehealth has benefitted care through enhanced monitoring, intervention, and self-care. Monitoring via wearable devices has improved proactive disease management of a diverse set of disorders; for example, when escalating care for postconcussive syndrome.[28] Mobile applications have also provided

Table 1
Capabilities of telehealth for patients and providers

Patient to provider	Synchronous (Videoconferencing, Instant Messaging)	Asynchronous (Store and Forward)	Continuous (Wearable Devices, Mobile Applications)
Patient-to-provider	• Live-interactive patient visits (such as virtual urgent care)	• Virtual chronic disease management • Virtual second opinion (such as grand rounds)	• Objective monitoring devices (such as Fitbit, Apple Watch) • Management tools (such as for asthma)
Provider-to-provider	• Live-interactive "curbside consult" • Telementoring (such as Project ECHO)	• eConsult (such as MSF Tele-Expertise) • eReferral (such as Champlain BASE)	—

	Synchronous (Video-conferencing, instant messaging)	Asynchronous (store-and-forward)	Continuous (Wearable devices, mobile applications)
Patient-to-provider	• Live-interactive patient visits (such as virtual urgent care)	• Virtual chronic disease management • Virtual "second opinion" (such as Grand Rounds)	• Objective monitoring devices (such as Fitbit, Apple Watch) • Management tools (such as for asthma)
Provider-to-provider	• Live-interactive "curbside consult" • Tele-mentoring (such as Project ECHO)	• eConsult (such as MSF Tele-Expertise) • eReferral (such as Champlain BASE)	

Provider to provider

Dimension	Description
Race/Ethnicity	White, African-American, Latin-American, etc...
Gender	Male, Female, Non-Binary, Transitioned, etc...
Sexual Identity	LGBTQ, etc...
Language	English, Spanish, Mandarin, Cantonese, etc...
Socioeconomic Status	By quintile, relative to federal poverty line
Insurance Coverage	Extent of cost-sharing, benefits, etc...
Geography	Zip code density, rural vs. urban
Modality	Power grid, cellular network, internet modem, software, hardware

Abbreviation: MSF, Médecins Sans Frontières.

Data from Delaigue S, Bonnardot L, Steichen O, et al. Seven years of telemedicine in Medecins Sans Frontieres demonstrate that offering direct specialist expertise in the frontline brings clinical and educational value. J Glob Health. 2018;8(2):020414.

platforms for care enhancement over the long term through regular notifications pushed by providers to patients; for instance, in the setting of asthma.[29] Self-care has been empowered by these sorts of modalities, through heightened proactive behaviors and engagement with health care in 89% and 83% of patients, according to a recent meta-analysis.[30]

However, the potential for IGIs is borne out of the nonrepresentativeness of most telehealth studies across several dimensions (**Table 2**). One such dimension is population representativeness. A recent review by Fiks and colleagues[31] found that the number of white people enrolled in studies for telehealth was double that of nonwhite populations. Another study found that Latino and Korean groups were 63% and 48% less likely to download health applications used for research than white cohorts.[32]

Furthermore, lack of representativeness bears downstream implications for these underserved cohorts. Data scientist Cathy O'Neil's[34] *Weapons of Math Destruction* and journalist Virginia Eubanks'[33] *Automating Inequality* both describe how using historically nonrepresentative data has unintentionally baked bias into algorithmic applications across disciplines (such as criminal justice sentencing and social services).[33,34] To the extent that telehealth datasets are used to train algorithms that diagnose and recommend treatments for diseases in the future, nonrepresentativeness can evolve into the inability to generalize these algorithms for populations excluded from telehealth.[35]

Excess Use and Cost of Care

The positive influence of telehealth on the cost of care delivery has also been noted. Over the short term, effects on inpatient use have included 72% fewer all-cause hospitalizations in CSHCN cohorts,[36] and effects on outpatient use have included 78% reductions in unnecessary face-to-face visits.[37] Over the long term, patients using dermatologic telehealth services had reduced use of follow-up and emergency care, leading to decreased costs of condition-specific care (such as psoriasis) of 45% over 6 months[38,39](**Fig. 2**). Across specialties, overall savings associated with direct medical expenditure reductions of up to 72% at payors (Aetna)[40] and integrated care systems (the Department of Veterans Affairs [VA]).[41]

Decreases in nonmedical costs have also been noted. In a study of publicly insured children in Georgia, indirect costs to families following introduction of telehealth services were one-third those before introduction.[42] At the VA, societal costs (including lost productivity) were reduced by 15% on introduction of telehealth modalities.[14,15,41]

States lead the rules for reimbursements and Medicaid in California (along with several other states) offers telehealth as a benefit. State laws are beginning to shift

| Table 2 | |
| **Dimensions of nonrepresentativeness relevant to telehealth** | |
Dimension	Description
Race/ethnicity	White, African American, Latin-American, and so forth
Gender	Male, female, nonbinary, transitioned, and so forth
Sexual identity	LGBTQ and so forth
Language	English, Spanish, Mandarin, Cantonese, and so forth
Socioeconomic status	By quintile, relative to federal poverty line
Insurance coverage	Extent of cost sharing, benefits, and so forth
Geography	Zip code density, rural vs urban
Modality	Power grid, cellular network, Internet modem, software, hardware

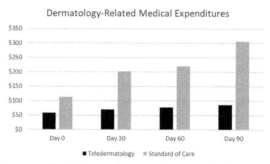

Fig. 2. Economic impacts of teledermatology on direct medical spending over 3 months. (*Data from* Snoswell CL, Caffery LJ, Whitty JA, et al. Cost-effectiveness of skin cancer referral and consultation using teledermoscopy in Australia. JAMA Dermatol. 2018;154(6):694-700.)

toward requiring all payers to cover telehealth services via the establishment of novel reimbursement codes.[43] However, until the rollout and adoption of such codes are more widespread, these innovative programs may only be available to families privately employed in organizations with robust corporate benefits and wellness plans.[24] In addition, although virtual visits can substitute for face-to-face visits, when virtual visits occur in addition to typical check-ups, and to the extent they trigger further referrals and/or testing, such supplementary care may not be covered by insurers. In vulnerable populations, additional out-of-pocket costs (exacerbated by increasing insurance cost sharing[44]) consume a disproportionate fraction of family wealth[45] (**Fig. 3**).

Access to Care

Telehealth is a key strategy to improve access within pediatric specialty care. Various modalities, including e-mail, store and forward, and real-time video, have all promoted the ability of populations under study to receive care services across specialties.[39,41,46] One particularly notable example is the Expanding Capacity for

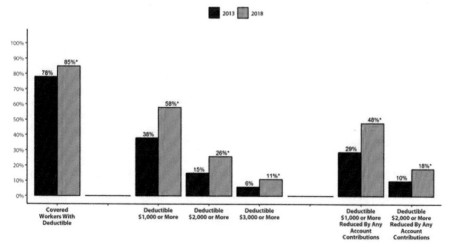

Fig. 3. Trends in deductible insurance plans and amount of deductibles, 2013 to 2018.* Statistical significance, p<0.05. (*From* Kaiser Family Foundation. Employer Health Benefits Survey. 2018. Available at: https://www.kff.org/report-section/2018-employer-health-benefits-survey-summary-of-findings/. Accessed September 30th, 2019; with permission.)

Healthcare Organizations (ECHO) initiative, which has promoted the delivery of complex care to niche cohorts (such adults with hepatitis C and children with autism).[6,47]

In addition, telehealth has shortened the time frame to the receipt of specialty care.[48] For safety-net populations in Los Angeles, California, response times decreased from 9 months to a median of 1 day.[49] Similar achievements exist in pediatric populations, including in high-risk cohorts such as neonates with very low birthweight, infants with cystic fibrosis, and teenagers with sickle cell anemia.[50–53] These technologies have also markedly improved access to ancillary care services, including nutrition, psychological, language interpretation, and remote home monitoring.[54]

However, opportunities exist to improve access more equally between populations. Another dimension of nonrepresentativeness relates to language, which fundamentally affects access (see **Table 1**).[55] For example, although fewer than half of all patients in a diverse urban cohort reported English as their primary language, non-English speakers are not specifically targeted in major digital technology ownership and usage surveys.[32] As a result, health care systems have not established technologies to serve these patients: 1 study found that, even in densely Spanish-speaking regions, only 45% of hospital technology platforms provided Spanish translations.[56]

Modality nonrepresentativeness also begets access disparities. Considerable differences exist in the hardware, software, modems, and networks to which separate populations have access, a phenomenon that has been termed the digital divide[2,57–61] (**Box 1**).

For example, a 2013 study found that Latin Americans were 19%, 29%, and 56% less likely than index groups to own smartphones, computers, and tablets, respectively.[32] Other considerations, such as power and cellular grids, may also exacerbate

---

Box 1
The digital divide in technological access between populations

The digital divide was first coined in a 1999 report by the US Department of Communications' National Telecommunications and Information Administration. At the time, African American and Latin-American households were 60% less likely to have Internet access, rural residents were 50% less likely than urban residents, the poor were up to 95% less likely than those in the highest income quartile, and those without a high school degree were 10% less likely than high school graduates (**Fig. 4**).

More recent studies have confirmed these disparities at new technological frontiers. The 2018 data from the National Technology Information Agency (NTIA) found that African American and Latin-American households were 10% less likely to use any form of Internet, 10% less likely to use smartphones, 30% to 39% less likely to use tablets, and 34% to 49% less likely to use wearables than white populations. The Pew Research Center's Mobile Technology and Home Broadband 2019 report found similar patterns when stratifying by geography, income, and education. For example, individuals with a high school education or less were 20% and 36% less likely to use smartphones and have access to home broadband, respectively.

Telehealth tools are frequently embedded across this variety of technologies, which can produce marked disparities in use. Recent NTIA data showed that minority, rural, and poor populations were nearly 30%, 33%, and 52% less likely to communicate with their doctors online or use online health monitoring services, respectively (**Fig. 5**). Simultaneously, Pew found that black and Hispanic populations are half as likely as white populations to use nonsmartphone forms of telehealth technologies. Individuals with low levels of income and education were found to be one-fourth as likely to use these alternative forms of technology compared with the index cohorts for which such inventions are typically designed.

Thus, failing to consider the digital divide can intensify what has been deemed a looming health care "apartheid."

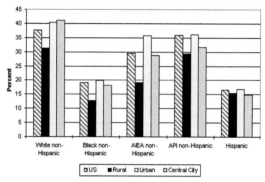

Fig. 4. Percentage of US persons using the Internet from any location, in 1998. AIEA, American Indian, Eskimo, or Aleut; API, Asian or Pacific Islander. (*From* National Technology Information Agency. Falling through the net: defining the digital divide. 1999. Available from: https://www.ntia.doc.gov/legacy/ntiahome/fttn99/contents.html. Accessed September 30th, 2019.)

access disparities in specific neighborhoods and regions, both domestically and internationally (**Fig. 6**).

Another cause of access disparities relates to systematic biases intrinsic to the health care system. Previous evidence has documented differences in access to care by minority groups to referral-sensitive conditions/procedures (such as colonoscopy and mammography)[62] and pain management.[63] Similarly, per 1 study, African Americans and Hispanic patients were 37.5% and 25% less likely to be issued access codes to hospital-affiliated telehealth technologies.[64]

IMPACTS OF TELEHEALTH ON A QUINTUPLE AIM FOR PEDIATRIC CARE

Beyond the Triple Aim, for optimal and equitable expansion of telehealth in pediatric care, 2 other principles must be adopted: impacts on the workforce, and implications on equity.

Workforce

Various studies have reported the positive influences of telehealth on the pediatric workforce, primarily by means of resolving unnecessary appointments, facilitating continuity of care, and enabling primary care provider (PCP) cross-training.

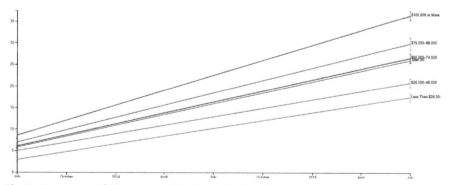

Fig. 5. Percentage of US persons using the online health monitoring services in 2015. (*From* Data Explorer: National Technology Information Agency. Available at: https://www.ntia.doc.gov/data/digital-nation-data-explorer#sel=internetUser&disp=map. Accessed September 30th, 2019.)

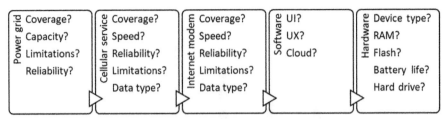

Fig. 6. Modality considerations for telehealth.UI, user interface; UX, user experience; RAM, random access memory.

1. Appointment resolution: at San Francisco General Hospital, the percentage of referrals made without a clear consultative question decreased by 44% and 75% in the medical and surgical specialty clinics, respectively, following introduction of a telehealth consultation tool.[65] Similarly, a Canadian e-consultation tool led to as much as 40% reductions in face-to-face referrals,[66] and increased resolution of cases by PCPs by 36%[67](**Fig. 7**).

2. Continuity of care: school-based telemedicine programs pioneered through the University of Rochester increased contact with children and adolescents not otherwise receiving primary care, leading to 54% reductions in school absences because of illness.[68]

3. PCP cross-training and peer-to-peer support: telementoring and information sharing have shown improved management of specialty issues by PCPs[20,47,67,69](**Fig. 8**). For example, 1 trial showed noninferior treatment protocols and outcomes compared with academic medical centers.[69] Similar findings have been documented at the University of California, San Francisco, and also in MSF cohorts, where marked decreases in changes in initial case management of

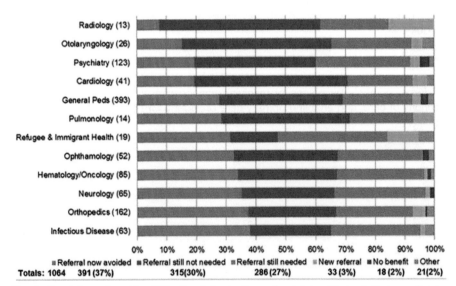

Fig. 7. Need for referral by PCP after introduction of a telehealth tool. Peds, pediatrics. (*From* Lai L, Liddy C, Keely E, et al. The impact of electronic consultation on a Canadian tertiary care pediatric specialty referral system: A prospective single-center observational study. PLoS One. 2018;13(1):e0190247.)

specialty issues handled by PCPs were noted following introduction of telehealth technologies.[26]

4. Work scheduling: because, by definition, telehealth technologies may be used remotely and in mobile settings, and because asynchronous applications grant time flexibility, providers and staff may arrange their schedules in keeping with personal preferences/needs.

Negative consequences imposed on the workforce by telehealth must be considered as well. Electronic health record technologies have been noted to "impos[e] an exhausting litany of clerical tasks for the clinical staff, contributing to staff burnout and waste" in academic and public health care settings.[70,71] If decentralized telehealth data need to be exported manually into hospital documentation, similar consequences could emerge related to burnout. Given lower staffing ratios at facilities serving minority and rural populations historically, amplification of burnout in these settings would affect care disproportionately.[72]

Equity

This last tier of the quintuple aim demands that technologies have comparable social outcomes between populations. Concerns related to equity primarily orbit around privacy and security considerations associated with the potential leakage of personalized health information (PHI).

Transmission of PHI is intrinsic to the value proposition of telehealth tools. However, neither iOS nor Android virtual stores have explicit policies addressing the privacy of PHI for the rapidly proliferating ranks of telehealth mobile apps housed within them.[73] Furthermore, in a review of the 600 most commonly used telehealth apps, only 31%

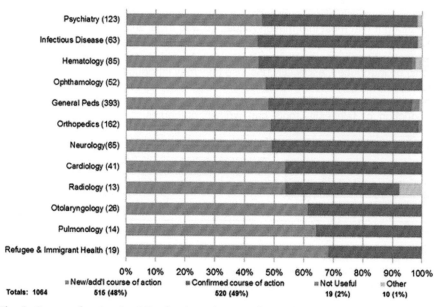

Fig. 8. Course of action by PCP after introduction of a telehealth tool. add'l, additional. (*From* Lai L, Liddy C, Keely E, et al. The impact of electronic consultation on a Canadian tertiary care pediatric specialty referral system: A prospective single-center observational study. PLoS One. 2018;13(1):e0190247.)

had any privacy policy.[74] Compounding the issue, the average reading grade level (RGL) of these apps was grade 12.8 (ie, beyond high school) for those explicitly targeting pediatric populations, considerably more than the average adult RGL of 8.0.[74]

Meanwhile, a separate review found that 64% and 82% of medical telehealth apps were sending unencrypted data over the Internet and using third-party storage and hosting services, respectively.[75] A stress-testing study revealed that 96% of telehealth apps posed some potential damage through security and privacy deficits, and 1 in 12 imposed the highest potential damages.[76] These sorts of security breaches leading to compromise of PHI may bear discriminatory consequences in the workplace or elsewhere, especially within populations unaware of how their data might be used or shared in the first place.[77]

GUIDING PRINCIPLES TO RESPONSIBLY IMPLEMENTING TELEHEALTH IN PEDIATRICS

As described by Veinot and colleagues,[24] "[a]n intervention produces inequality if it is (a) more accessible to, (b) adopted more frequently by, (c) adhered to more closely by, or (d) more effective in socioeconomically advantaged groups." Ten factors important to ensure the equitable and responsible implementation of telehealth in pediatrics are highlighted here (**Fig. 9**).

Judiciousness

Developers of telehealth technologies must ensure that their tools produce material progress for patient care. Although so-called big data are an asset that technology developers can use, invocations for meaningful use of PHI must likewise apply to the use of large datasets in telehealth.[78] In contrast, the capacity for telehealth technologies to generate voluminous data is not normatively useful (generation of PHI is justifiable only when it is impactful) and thus the sourcing of data must also be meaningful.[79] For example, appraisals of diabetes self-care apps have found that patients and providers alike thought that most information requested was trivial and not useful.[80]

Considering telehealth through both a meaningful sourcing and using framework implies that just because new tools are technically feasible to create does not mean they should be introduced, especially because they may introduce new layers of administrative complexity to the care process.[81] This point is especially true in the setting of direct-to-consumer (DTC) apps, which can further fragment care.[82] In these scenarios, introduction of telehealth tools can worsen outcomes: 1 study found that DTC

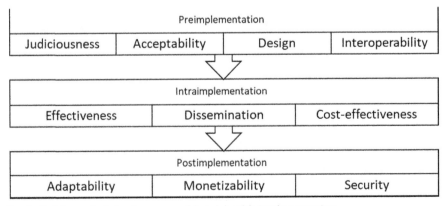

Fig. 9. Guiding principles for responsible telehealth implementation.

telemedicine users were 70% and 11% more likely to have urgent care and emergency department visits over 5 years compared with nonusers.[83]

Acceptability

Telehealth tools must be acceptable across populations. Ethnographic study can educate developers on prerequisite considerations to use in various populations. For example, a study on the adoption of telehealth at Kaiser Permanente found that elderly Latin Americans and African Americans were 43% and 32% less likely to desire video visits compared with face-to-face ones (even when unnecessary).[84] Other studies have found increased fear of erosion of existing personal relationships with providers associated with telehealth tools in these populations.[85]

Resistance to telehealth in specific populations may also be rooted in negative historical experiences (such as Tuskegee for African American populations), leading to poor perceptions of unfamiliar medical technologies.[85,86] Increasing levels of mistrust have been correlated with 56%, 48%, and 11% increased risk of nonadherence to medical advice, prescriptions, and follow-up care, respectively.[87,88] Using hospital family advisory councils and focus groups can help decipher the acceptability of a telehealth program across multiple cultures and histories.

Design

Keen attention to the design of telehealth tools can increase uptake by both patients and providers through regular usability analyses (these are only conducted by 34% of studies per 1 review).[30] Elements of design can address issues related to technological anxiety, self-efficacy, perceived usefulness, ease of use, intent to use, and use behaviors[89](**Fig. 10**). For example, 1 study found that patients with very limited health literacy required up to 4 times longer to complete tasks with an app for diabetes, and another found that minority patients could not complete up to 57% of required tasks.[90,91] Comprehensive design decisions have been shown to improve adoption of new health care technologies.[92]

As such, codesign with patients can lead to increased relevance, greater engagement, and more rapid uptake of new tools.[89] Decisions related to inclusive design can be particularly important for medically disabled groups.[24] Contextual study

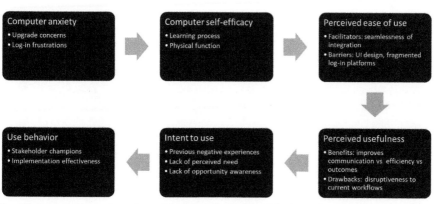

Fig. 10. Design elements and considerations for telehealth. (*Data from* Unertl KM, Schaefbauer CL, Campbell TR, et al. Integrating community-based participatory research and informatics approaches to improve the engagement and health of underserved populations. J Am Med Inform Assoc. 2016;23(1):60-73.)

methods, such as community-based participatory research, can both reveal barriers to uptake and leverage resources for uptake.[89] Analogously, codesign with providers, especially when focusing on integration with workflows and compatibility with technological infrastructure, has been shown to increase clinical engagement.[80,81,93]

Interoperability

Interoperability, both within and between institutions, is foundational for the longer-term usefulness of telehealth. Presently, most health record data are institution specific, and fewer than one-third of hospitals are capable of (1) finding, (2) sending, (3) receiving, and (4) integrating electronic information from outside providers.[94]

Without interoperability, data streams from telehealth tools are likely to remain sequestered, creating silos of small data rather than warehouses of big data.[95,96] As a result, up to three-quarters of electronic infrastructure costs have been devoted to troubleshooting idiosyncratic protocols of numerous, independent technologies via so-called middleware, all of which results in limited usability for patient care[70,97] (**Fig. 11**).

Guidelines for standardization across levels of patient care have been put forth by the National Academy of Medicine's 2019 *Procuring Interoperability* report, and these should be consulted by developers (before production) and health systems (before investment and implementation).[98] Technical and syntactic standards exist to promote an open-source, modular ecosystem of telehealth applications (rather than walled-off, proprietary systems).[95,96,99] In this way, interoperability can empower telehealth to capitalize on the opportunity to solve care delivery challenges that the current in-person care has not been able to solve to date.

Effectiveness

Individual and population-level impacts should be considered to further close the gap in real-world effectiveness of telehealth between cohorts.

On an individual level, the following characteristics affect the ability to receive care via telehealth modalities: literacy, numeracy, self-efficacy, and engagement.[65,100,101] Historically, trials have enrolled predominantly patients who are engaged in their

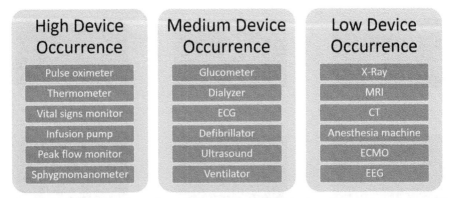

Fig. 11. Examples of independent data-collecting technologies at the point of care. CT, computed tomography; ECG, electrocardiogram; ECMO, extracorporeal membrane oxygenation; EEG, electroencephalogram. (*Data from* Cantwell E, McDermott K. making technology talk: how interoperability can improve care, drive efficiency, and reduce waste. Healthc Financ Manage. 2016;70(5):70-6.)

own health care (62% of those studied, per 1 review) and with a postgraduate education (86% of those enrolled).[31] From the individual provider perspective, technical literacy and self-efficacy are also critical, as are clinical contextual factors (such as staffing resource availability) that may be missing in facilities serving vulnerable populations.[102,103]

At the population level, adequate credentialing is necessary to ensure universally effective care, but 1 study found that only 26% of dermatology encounters across 16 DTC sites disclosed licensure (and several of these lacked appropriate licensing).[93] In turn, protocols can ensure adequate communication of potential harms related to recommended care (the same study showed relevant adverse effects were disclosed in only 32% of encounters).[93] In addition, because data generated by telehealth technologies form the pipeline for future research, recruitment methods that leverage these tools for demographic inclusivity can promote a positive feedback loop for effectiveness[104–107] (**Box 2**).

Dissemination

A place-based approach to dissemination of telehealth technologies can stimulate uptake across populations. The manner and media of dissemination should be considerate of contextual social factors.[108] For example, to inform its place-based approach, the Bay Area Regional Health Inequalities Initiative includes living conditions as a prominent consideration in its framework for reconciling outcomes gaps.[109] Telehealth tools should be validated for practicality and usefulness in these settings. Moreover, in the future, these technologies could provide a more nuanced approach to screening of social determinants of health, providing a self-reinforcing evidence pipeline.[110]

Cost-Effectiveness

To support the sustainability of telehealth, attention must be paid to the financial appraisal of these technologies. At present, there is a lack of clarity around the reimbursement processes for telehealth tools, a dimension of uncertainty that limits the feasibility of deploying these technologies in lower-resource settings,[54] especially given the high upfront costs of infrastructure to support telehealth: from surveys of a pediatric telehealth research network, 38% and 66% of responding programs reported investments greater than $1 million and $100,000, respectively.[54] Because 85% of programs reported institutional dollars as the primary source of funding, cost-effectiveness is especially critical in systems with tighter budgetary constraints.[54] The cost-effectiveness of telehealth should also be compared with alternative proven interventions to render the greatest impact from the societal perspective.[39,41,111]

Box 2
Use of telehealth technologies to promote inclusive research

Inclusive research can help avoid the sort of excessive homogeneity that causes failure in external validation and leads to an inability to generalize. Telehealth tools offer an opportunity to increase recruitment in settings that may have been excluded or avoided previously.

In 1 standout example, Davis and colleagues[106] leveraged videoconferencing to recruit patients to a diabetes self-management study from 3 community health centers located more than 160 km (100 miles) from the primary academic medical center site in South Carolina. In another, a London-based study team used videoconferencing to enroll patients to a study evaluating the efficacy of glaucoma radiation therapy across 3 regions in South Africa.

Adaptability

Patient engagement has been described as the "blockbuster drug of the 21st century."[112] It is incumbent on developers and implementers to harness this potential by setting up feedback loops through which telehealth engagement can be monitored, evaluated, and improved on.[113] To cultivate a cycle of continuous learning, assessment dashboards should incorporate engagement metrics beyond outcomes alone, as has been pioneered in a consortium of pain clinics across Ontario[114](**Fig. 12**). Subjective dashboards, such as the VA's Customer Experience Analytics suite, can also solicit opportunities for improvement that can be systematically addressed in subsequent versions of the technology.[115,116]

Monetizability

State policies vary on the reimbursement level around telehealth. Centers for Medicare & Medicaid Services, Health & Human Services, and state laws all vary on what is reimbursable. This vagueness leads to confusion by health systems related to how to implement telehealth in fiscally responsible ways to patients. As many health systems consider how to justify implementing and offering telehealth to their patients in a sustainable manner, there is a large role for state and national advocacy to promote equal reimbursement for telehealth serving Medicaid and vulnerable population groups. In addition, insofar as telehealth tools may be profit generating for their developers and/or implementing institutions, regulatory action must protect participating patients from exploitation. Consent processes should clearly communicate any possible financial gains harvested from patient data.[77] Clarity in this communication can promote patient trust that fosters the uptake of these technologies and thereby enables the improvement of health in the long-term.

Security

In addition, as touched on in the previous discussion of equity, considerations of privacy, security, confidentiality, and anonymity are fundamental to the responsible

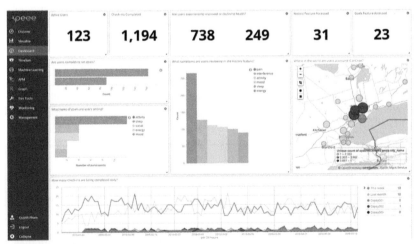

Fig. 12. Sample characteristics of objective engagement dashboards. (*From* Pham Q, Graham G, Lalloo C, et al. An analytics platform to evaluate effective engagement with pediatric mobile health apps: design, development, and formative evaluation. JMIR Mhealth Uhealth. 2018;6(12):e11447.)

implementation of telehealth in pediatrics. Reidentification of PHI, third-party information sharing, and data breaches that expose already-vulnerable groups can worsen trust and participation in the health care system by these populations over the long run.[33,34,117] Codified authorization protocols for sharing of PHI must be adopted and the development of governance technologies must be prioritized going forward.[95,99,118,119]

HOW CAN THE EXPANSION OF TELEHEALTH IN PEDIATRICS BE SUPPORTED?

In conclusion, telehealth can revolutionize the delivery of pediatric care. However, all stakeholders (patients, providers, health care systems, health information technology developers (both incumbent and startup), payors, and policymakers) must play a role to ensure that these improvements are equitable across populations. Through inclusive research, collaborative design, continuous communication, considerate implementation, comprehensive regulation, and rapid iteration, these stakeholders can promote the achievement of a quintuple aim for telehealth serving children.

DISCLOSURE

S. Thadaney-Israni serves on the board of Scients.org, for which she receives no remuneration. The remaining authors have nothing to disclose.

REFERENCES

1. Berwick DM, Nolan TW, Whittington J. The triple aim: care, health, and cost. Health Aff (Millwood) 2008;27(3):759–69.
2. AI in healthcare: the hope, the hype, the promise, the peril. National Academy of Medicine; 2019. Available at: https://nam.edu/wp-content/uploads/2019/12/AI-in-Health-Care-PREPUB-FINAL.pdf.
3. Bethell CD, Kogan MD, Strickland BB, et al. A national and state profile of leading health problems and health care quality for US children: key insurance disparities and across-state variations. Acad Pediatr 2011;11(3 Suppl):S22–33.
4. Committee on Hospital Care and Institute for Patient- and Family-Centered Care. Patient- and family-centered care and the pediatrician's role. Pediatrics 2012; 129(2):394–404.
5. Coker TR, Rodriguez MA, Flores G. Family-centered care for US children with special health care needs: who gets it and why? Pediatrics 2010;125(6): 1159–67.
6. Mazurek MO, Brown R, Curran A, et al. ECHO Autism. Clin Pediatr (Phila) 2017; 56(3):247–56.
7. Marcin JP, Ellis J, Mawis R, et al. Using telemedicine to provide pediatric subspecialty care to children with special health care needs in an underserved rural community. Pediatrics 2004;113(1 Pt 1):1–6.
8. Mayer ML. Are we there yet? Distance to care and relative supply among pediatric medical subspecialties. Pediatrics 2006;118(6):2313–21.
9. Mayer ML. Disparities in geographic access to pediatric subspecialty care. Matern Child Health J 2008;12(5):624–32.
10. Clemans-Cope L, Kenney G, Waidmann T, et al. How Well Is CHIP Addressing Health Care Access and Affordability for Children? Acad Pediatr 2015;15(3 Suppl):S71–7.

11. Ireys HT, Anderson GF, Shaffer TJ, et al. Expenditures for care of children with chronic illnesses enrolled in the Washington State Medicaid program, fiscal year 1993. Pediatrics 1997;100(2 Pt 1):197–204.

12. Cohen E, Berry JG, Camacho X, et al. Patterns and costs of health care use of children with medical complexity. Pediatrics 2012;130(6):e1463–70.

13. Berry JG, Hall M, Neff J, et al. Children with medical complexity and Medicaid: spending and cost savings. Health Aff (Millwood) 2014;33(12):2199–206.

14. McCormick MC, Bernbaum JC, Eisenberg JM, et al. Costs incurred by parents of very low birth weight infants after the initial neonatal hospitalization. Pediatrics 1991;88(3):533–41.

15. Bloom BS, Knorr RS, Evans AE. The epidemiology of disease expenses. The costs of caring for children with cancer. JAMA 1985;253(16):2393–7.

16. Committee On Pediatric W, Marcin JP, Rimsza ME, et al. The use of telemedicine to address access and physician workforce shortages. Pediatrics 2015;136(1): 202–9.

17. Ray KN, Kahn JM. Connected subspecialty care: applying telehealth strategies to specific referral barriers. Acad Pediatr 2020;20(1):16–22.

18. Chen AH, Murphy EJ, Yee HF Jr. eReferral–a new model for integrated care. N Engl J Med 2013;368(26):2450–3.

19. Medical Home Initiatives for Children With Special Needs Project Advisory Committee. American Academy of Pediatrics. The medical home. Pediatrics 2002; 110(1 Pt 1):184–6.

20. Delaigue S, Bonnardot L, Steichen O, et al. Seven years of telemedicine in Medecins Sans Frontieres demonstrate that offering direct specialist expertise in the frontline brings clinical and educational value. J Glob Health 2018;8(2): 020414.

21. Turley M, Garrido T, Lowenthal A, et al. Association between personal health record enrollment and patient loyalty. Am J Manag Care 2012;18(7):e248–53.

22. Tieu L, Sarkar U, Schillinger D, et al. Barriers and facilitators to online portal use among patients and caregivers in a safety net health care system: a qualitative study. J Med Internet Res 2015;17(12):e275.

23. Featherall J, Lapin B, Chaitoff A, et al. Characterization of patient interest in provider-based consumer health information technology: survey study. J Med Internet Res 2018;20(4):e128.

24. Veinot TC, Mitchell H, Ancker JS. Good intentions are not enough: how informatics interventions can worsen inequality. J Am Med Inform Assoc 2018; 25(8):1080–8.

25. Martinez Garcia D, Bonnardot L, Olson D, et al. A retrospective analysis of pediatric cases handled by the MSF tele-expertise system. Front Public Health 2014;2:266.

26. Zachariah R, Bienvenue B, Ayada L, et al. Practicing medicine without borders: tele-consultations and tele-mentoring for improving paediatric care in a conflict setting in Somalia? Trop Med Int Health 2012;17(9):1156–62.

27. Dayal P, Hojman NM, Kissee JL, et al. Impact of telemedicine on severity of illness and outcomes among children transferred from referring emergency departments to a Children's Hospital PICU. Pediatr Crit Care Med 2016;17(6): 516–21.

28. Huber DL, Thomas DG, Danduran M, et al. Quantifying activity levels after sport-related concussion using actigraph and mobile (mHealth) technologies. J Athl Train 2019;54(9):929–38.

29. Mammen JR, Java JJ, Halterman J, et al. Development and preliminary results of an Electronic Medical Record (EMR)-integrated smartphone telemedicine program to deliver asthma care remotely. J Telemed Telecare 2019. 1357633X19870025. Available at: https://www.ncbi.nlm.nih.gov/pubmed/31438761.

30. Sawesi S, Rashrash M, Phalakornkule K, et al. The impact of information technology on patient engagement and health behavior change: a systematic review of the literature. JMIR Med Inform 2016;4(1):e1.

31. Fiks AG, Fleisher L, Berrigan L, et al. Usability, acceptability, and impact of a pediatric teledermatology mobile health application. Telemed J E Health 2018; 24(3):236–45.

32. Bender MS, Choi J, Arai S, et al. Digital technology ownership, usage, and factors predicting downloading health apps among caucasian, filipino, korean, and latino americans: the digital link to health survey. JMIR Mhealth Uhealth 2014; 2(4):e43.

33. Eubanks V. Automating inequality : how high-tech tools profile, police, and punish the poor. First Edition. New York: St. Martin's Press; 2017. p. 260.

34. O'Neil C. Weapons of math destruction : how big data increases inequality and threatens democracy. New York: Crown Publishers; 2016.

35. Cahan EM, Hernandez-Boussard T, Thadaney-Israni S, et al. Putting the data before the algorithm in big data addressing personalized healthcare. NPJ Digit Med 2019;2:78.

36. Dayal P, Chang CH, Benko WS, et al. Hospital utilization among rural children served by pediatric neurology telemedicine clinics. JAMA Netw Open 2019; 2(8):e199364.

37. Marcolino MS, Pereira Afonso dos Santos J, Santos Neves D, et al. Teleconsultations to provide support for primary care practitioners and improve quality of care–the experience of a large scale telehealth service in Brazil. Stud Health Technol Inform 2015;216:987.

38. Parsi MA, Ellis JJ, Lashner BA. Cost-effectiveness of quantitative fecal lactoferrin assay for diagnosis of symptomatic patients with ileal pouch-anal anastomosis. J Clin Gastroenterol 2008;42(7):799–805.

39. Snoswell CL, Caffery LJ, Whitty JA, et al. Cost-effectiveness of skin cancer referral and consultation using teledermoscopy in Australia. JAMA Dermatol 2018;154(6):694–700.

40. Rajda J, Seraly MP, Fernandes J, et al. Impact of direct to consumer store-and-forward teledermatology on access to care, satisfaction, utilization, and costs in a commercial health plan population. Telemed J E Health 2018;24(2):166–9.

41. Datta SK, Warshaw EM, Edison KE, et al. Cost and utility analysis of a store-and-forward teledermatology referral system: a randomized clinical trial. JAMA Dermatol 2015;151(12):1323–9.

42. Karp WB, Grigsby RK, McSwiggan-Hardin M, et al. Use of telemedicine for children with special health care needs. Pediatrics 2000;105(4 Pt 1):843–7.

43. Daniel JG, Uppaluru M. New reimbursement for remote patient monitoring and telemedicine: crowell and moring. Available at: https://www.cmhealthlaw.com/2017/11/new-reimbursement-for-remote-patient-monitoring-and-telemedicine/. Accessed November 3, 2017.

44. Employer health benefits survey. Kaiser Family Foundation; 2018. Available at: https://www.kff.org/report-section/2018-employer-health-benefits-survey-summary-of-findings/.

45. Lewey J, Gagne JJ, Franklin J, et al. Impact of high deductible health plans on cardiovascular medication adherence and health disparities. Circ Cardiovasc Qual Outcomes 2018;11(11):e004632.

46. Snoswell C, Finnane A, Janda M, et al. Cost-effectiveness of store-and-forward teledermatology: a systematic review. JAMA Dermatol 2016;152(6):702–8.

47. Arora S, Thornton K, Murata G, et al. Outcomes of treatment for hepatitis C virus infection by primary care providers. N Engl J Med 2011;364(23):2199–207.

48. Bonnardot L, Liu J, Wootton E, et al. The development of a multilingual tool for facilitating the primary-specialty care interface in low resource settings: the MSF tele-expertise system. Front Public Health 2014;2:126.

49. Barnett ML, Yee HF Jr, Mehrotra A, et al. Los Angeles safety-net program econsult system was rapidly adopted and decreased wait times to see specialists. Health Aff (Millwood) 2017;36(3):492–9.

50. Madu PN, Chang AY, Kayembe MK, et al. Teledermatology as a means to provide multispecialty care: a case of global specialty collaboration. Pediatr Dermatol 2017;34(2):e89–92.

51. Gray JE, Safran C, Davis RB, et al. Baby CareLink: using the internet and telemedicine to improve care for high-risk infants. Pediatrics 2000;106(6):1318–24.

52. Martinez-Millana A, Zettl A, Floch J, et al. The Potential of Self-Management mHealth for Pediatric Cystic Fibrosis: Mixed-Methods Study for Health Care and App Assessment. JMIR Mhealth Uhealth 2019;7(4):e13362.

53. Badawy SM. iManage: A novel self-management app for sickle cell disease. Pediatr Blood Cancer 2017;64(5).

54. Olson CA, McSwain SD, Curfman AL, et al. The current pediatric telehealth landscape. Pediatrics 2018;141(3) [pii:e20172334].

55. Sadasivaiah S, Lyles CR, Kiyoi S, et al. Disparities in patient-reported interest in web-based patient portals: survey at an urban academic safety-net hospital. J Med Internet Res 2019;21(3):e11421.

56. Gallant LM, Irizarry C, Boone GM, et al. Spanish content on hospital websites: an analysis of U.S. Hospitals' in concentrated Latino communities. J Comput Mediat Commun 2010;15(4):552–74.

57. Gibbons MC. A historical overview of health disparities and the potential of eHealth solutions. J Med Internet Res 2005;7(5):e50.

58. Falling through the net: defining the digital divide: National Technology Information Agency (NTIA). 1999. Available at: https://www.ntia.doc.gov/legacy/ntiahome/fttn99/contents.html.

59. Data explorer: National Technology Information Agency. Available at: https://www.ntia.doc.gov/data/digital-nation-data-explorer#sel=internetUser&disp=map.

60. Irizarry T, DeVito Dabbs A, Curran CR. Patient portals and patient engagement: a state of the science review. J Med Internet Res 2015;17(6):e148.

61. Pew Research Center. Mobile technology and home broadband 2019 2019.

62. McBean AM, Gornick M. Differences by race in the rates of procedures performed in hospitals for Medicare beneficiaries. Health Care Financ Rev 1994;15(4):77–90.

63. Hoffman KM, Trawalter S, Axt JR, et al. Racial bias in pain assessment and treatment recommendations, and false beliefs about biological differences between blacks and whites. Proc Natl Acad Sci U S A 2016;113(16):4296–301.

64. Ancker JS, Barron Y, Rockoff ML, et al. Use of an electronic patient portal among disadvantaged populations. J Gen Intern Med 2011;26(10):1117–23.

65. Liddy C, Moroz I, Mihan A, et al. A systematic review of asynchronous, provider-to-provider, electronic consultation services to improve access to specialty care available worldwide. Telemed J E Health 2019;25(3):184–98.
66. Keely E, Liddy C, Afkham A. Utilization, benefits, and impact of an e-consultation service across diverse specialties and primary care providers. Telemed J E Health 2013;19(10):733–8.
67. Lai L, Liddy C, Keely E, et al. The impact of electronic consultation on a Canadian tertiary care pediatric specialty referral system: A prospective single-center observational study. PLoS One 2018;13(1):e0190247.
68. McConnochie KM, Wood NE, Kitzman HJ, et al. Telemedicine reduces absence resulting from illness in urban child care: evaluation of an innovation. Pediatrics 2005;115(5):1273–82.
69. Arora S, Kalishman S, Dion D, et al. Partnering urban academic medical centers and rural primary care clinicians to provide complex chronic disease care. Health Aff (Millwood) 2011;30(6):1176–84.
70. Cantwell E, McDermott K. making technology talk: how interoperability can improve care, drive effidcincy, and reduce waste. Healthc Financ Manage 2016;70(5):70–6.
71. Lee MS, Ray KN, Mehrotra A, et al. Primary Care Practitioners' Perceptions of Electronic Consult Systems: A Qualitative Analysis. JAMA Intern Med 2018; 178(6):782–9.
72. Kindig DA, Yan G. Physician supply in rural areas with large minority populations. Health Aff (Millwood) 1993;12(2):177–84.
73. Sunyaev A, Dehling T, Taylor PL, et al. Availability and quality of mobile health app privacy policies. J Am Med Inform Assoc 2015;22(e1):e28–33.
74. Das G, Cheung C, Nebeker C, et al. Privacy policies for apps targeted toward youth: descriptive analysis of readability. JMIR Mhealth Uhealth 2018;6(1):e3.
75. He D, Naveed M, Gunter CA, et al. Security concerns in Android mHealth Apps. AMIA Annu Symp Proc 2014;2014:645–54.
76. Dehling T, Gao F, Schneider S, et al. Exploring the far side of mobile health: information security and privacy of mobile health apps on iOS and Android. JMIR Mhealth Uhealth 2015;3(1):e8.
77. Cahan EM, H-BT, Thadaney-Israni S. Digital HeLa: ethical considerations for monetizable big data in healthcare. Nature Medicine, in press.
78. Chawla NV, Davis DA. Bringing big data to personalized healthcare: a patient-centered framework. J Gen Intern Med 2013;28(Suppl 3):S660–5.
79. Loscalzo J. Association studies in an era of too much information: clinical analysis of new biomarker and genetic data. Circulation 2007;116(17):1866–70.
80. Urowitz S, Wiljer D, Dupak K, et al. Improving diabetes management with a patient portal: a qualitative study of diabetes self-management portal. J Med Internet Res 2012;14(6):e158.
81. Vuononvirta T, Timonen M, Keinanen-Kiukaanniemi S, et al. The compatibility of telehealth with health-care delivery. J Telemed Telecare 2011;17(4):190–4.
82. Conners GP, Kressly SJ, Perrin JM, et al. Nonemergency acute care: when it's not the medical home. Pediatrics 2017;139(5) [pii:e20170629].
83. Ray KN, Shi Z, Poon SJ, et al. Use of commercial direct-to-consumer telemedicine by children. Acad Pediatr 2019;19(6):665–9.
84. Gordon NP, Hornbrook MC. Differences in access to and preferences for using patient portals and other eHealth technologies based on race, ethnicity, and age: a database and survey study of seniors in a large health plan. J Med Internet Res 2016;18(3):e50.

85. Lyles CR, Allen JY, Poole D, et al. "I want to keep the personal relationship with my doctor": understanding barriers to portal use among African Americans and Latinos. J Med Internet Res 2016;18(10):e263.

86. Corbie-Smith G, Thomas SB, Williams MV, et al. Attitudes and beliefs of African Americans toward participation in medical research. J Gen Intern Med 1999; 14(9):537–46.

87. Arnett MJ, Thorpe RJ Jr, Gaskin DJ, et al. Race, medical mistrust, and segregation in primary care as usual source of care: findings from the exploring health disparities in integrated communities study. J Urban Health 2016;93(3):456–67.

88. LaVeist TA, Isaac LA, Williams KP. Mistrust of health care organizations is associated with underutilization of health services. Health Serv Res 2009;44(6): 2093–105.

89. Unertl KM, Schaefbauer CL, Campbell TR, et al. Integrating community-based participatory research and informatics approaches to improve the engagement and health of underserved populations. J Am Med Inform Assoc 2016;23(1): 60–73.

90. Sarkar U, Gourley GI, Lyles CR, et al. Usability of commercially available mobile applications for diverse patients. J Gen Intern Med 2016;31(12):1417–26.

91. Tieu L, Schillinger D, Sarkar U, et al. Online patient websites for electronic health record access among vulnerable populations: portals to nowhere? J Am Med Inform Assoc 2017;24(e1):e47–54.

92. Portz JD, Bayliss EA, Bull S, et al. Using the technology acceptance model to explore user experience, intent to use, and use behavior of a patient portal among older adults with multiple chronic conditions: descriptive qualitative study. J Med Internet Res 2019;21(4):e11604.

93. Resneck JS Jr. Transparency associated with interactions between industry and physicians: deficits in accuracy and consistency of public data releases. JAMA Dermatol 2016;152(12):1303–4.

94. Holmgren AJ, Patel V, Adler-Milstein J. Progress in interoperability: measuring US hospitals' engagement in sharing patient data. Health Aff (Millwood) 2017; 36(10):1820–7.

95. Mandl KD, Mandel JC, Kohane IS. Driving innovation in health systems through an apps-based information economy. Cell Syst 2015;1(1):8–13.

96. Lehne M, Sass J, Essenwanger A, et al. Why digital medicine depends on interoperability. NPJ Digit Med 2019;2:79.

97. Gandhi R, Verma S, Baltassis E, et al. Look before you leap into the data lake. Boston Consulting Group; 2016. Available at: https://www.bcg.com/de-de/publications/2016/big-data-advanced-analytics-technology-digital-look-before-you-leap-into-data-lake.aspx.

98. Pronovost PJ, National Academy of Medicine (U.S.). Procuring interoperability : achieving high-quality, connected, and person-centered care. Washington, DC: NAM.EDU; 2018.

99. Mandl KD, Kohane IS. No small change for the health information economy. N Engl J Med 2009;360(13):1278–81.

100. Utidjian L, Abramson E. Pediatric Telehealth: Opportunities and Challenges. Pediatr Clin North Am 2016;63(2):367–78.

101. Ray KN, Ashcraft LE, Mehrotra A, et al. Family Perspectives on Telemedicine for Pediatric Subspecialty Care. Telemed J E Health 2017;23(10):852–62.

102. Rogove HJ, McArthur D, Demaerschalk BM, et al. Barriers to telemedicine: survey of current users in acute care units. Telemed J E Health 2012;18(1):48–53.

103. Broens TH, Huis in't Veld RM, Vollenbroek-Hutten MM, et al. Determinants of successful telemedicine implementations: a literature study. J Telemed Telecare 2007;13(6):303–9.
104. Burke BL Jr, Hall RW, Section on Telehealth Care. Telemedicine: pediatric applications. Pediatrics 2015;136(1):e293–308.
105. Sweeney TE, Haynes WA, Vallania F, et al. Methods to increase reproducibility in differential gene expression via meta-analysis. Nucleic Acids Res 2017; 45(1):e1.
106. Davis RM, Hitch AD, Nichols M, et al. A collaborative approach to the recruitment and retention of minority patients with diabetes in rural community health centers. Contemp Clin Trials 2009;30(1):63–70.
107. Kennedy C, Kirwan J, Cook C, et al. Telemedicine techniques can be used to facilitate the conduct of multicentre trials. J Telemed Telecare 2000;6(6):343–7 [discussion: 7-9].
108. Andrade EL, Evans WD, Barrett ND, et al. Development of the place-based Adelante social marketing campaign for prevention of substance use, sexual risk and violence among Latino immigrant youth. Health Educ Res 2018;33(2): 125–44.
109. Bay Area Regional Health Inequities Initiative (BARHII) Framework 2015. Available at: http://barhii.org/framework/.
110. Choi NG, Sirey JA, Bruce ML. Depression in homebound older adults: recent advances in screening and psychosocial interventions. Curr Transl Geriatr Exp Gerontol Rep 2013;2(1):16–23.
111. Khanal S, Burgon J, Leonard S, et al. Recommendations for the improved effectiveness and reporting of telemedicine programs in developing countries: results of a systematic literature review. Telemed J E Health 2015;21(11):903–15.
112. Kish L. The blockbuster drug of the century: an engaged patient: health standards. 2012. Available at: http://healthstandards.com/blog/2012/08/28/drug-of-the-century/.
113. Yardley L, Spring BJ, Riper H, et al. Understanding and promoting effective engagement with digital behavior change interventions. Am J Prev Med 2016; 51(5):833–42.
114. Pham Q, Graham G, Lalloo C, et al. An analytics platform to evaluate effective engagement with pediatric mobile health apps: design, development, and formative evaluation. JMIR Mhealth Uhealth 2018;6(12):e11447.
115. Nazi KM, Turvey CL, Klein DM, et al. A decade of veteran voices: examining patient portal enhancements through the lens of user-centered design. J Med Internet Res 2018;20(7):e10413.
116. Wootton R, Liu J, Bonnardot L. Assessing the quality of teleconsultations in a store-and-forward telemedicine network - long-term monitoring taking into account differences between cases. Front Public Health 2014;2:211.
117. Na LS, Yang C, Lo CC, et al. Feasibility of reidentifying individuals in large national physical activity data sets from which protected health information has been removed with use of machine learning. JAMA Netw Open 2018;1(8): e186040.
118. Mandl KD, Kohane IS. Time for a patient-driven health information economy? N Engl J Med 2016;374(3):205–8.
119. Cohen IG, Mello MM. Big data, big tech, and protecting patient privacy. JAMA 2019;322(12):1141–2.

Creating a Learning Televillage and Automated Digital Child Health Ecosystem

Ng Kee Chong, MBBS, MMed(Paeds), FAMS (Singapore), FRCPCH (UK), eMBA[a,*],
Chew Chu Shan Elaine, MBBS, MMed(Paeds), MRCPCh (UK), MCI[b],
Dirk F. de Korne, PhD, MSc[c,d,e]

KEYWORDS

- Child health • Internet of things in pediatrics • Big data
- Artificial intelligence (AI) in pediatrics • Population child health

KEY POINTS

- Automation is posed to transform many aspects of pediatrics.
- Automated digital health with the Internet of things will allow better collection of real-world data for generation of real-world evidence to improve child health.
- Population health science allows automated digital health and potentially reduces childhood obesity.
- Real-world data and real-world evidence using artificial intelligence allows development of a learning health system leading to a sustaining digital learning ecosystem for child health.

INTRODUCTION

The fourth industrial revolution promises to transform various aspects of social interaction, including pediatric health care. Telehealth was introduced 2 decades ago and although it initially faced resistance and cost barriers, it has increasingly shown evidence of improvement. Digitalization touches almost every aspect of care, including consultations bundled with the Internet of things (IoT), to enable more effective monitoring of patients and calibration of treatment. However, large-scale evidence from robust trials is currently lacking.

Increasingly, more cost-effective wireless technologies are focusing on patient and caregiver centeredness; for example, with apps that focus on child, parent, and

[a] Medical Innovation & Care Transformation, Division of Medicine, KK Women's & Children's Hospital, 100 Bukit Timah Road, Singapore 229899, Singapore; [b] Adolescent Medicine Service, Department of Paediatrics, KK Women's & Children's Hospital, Singapore; [c] Medical Innovation & Care Transformation, KK Women's & Children's Hospital, Singapore; [d] Erasmus School of Health Policy & Management, Erasmus University Rotterdam, Netherlands; [e] SVRZ Cares in Zeeland, Middelburg, Netherlands
* Corresponding author.
E-mail address: ng.kee.chong@singhealth.com.sg

Pediatr Clin N Am 67 (2020) 707–724
https://doi.org/10.1016/j.pcl.2020.04.016
0031-3955/20/© 2020 Elsevier Inc. All rights reserved.

clinician interactions and chatbots that allow patients to be digitally engaged with the clinic on a continuous basis. In addition, sensors in wearables create an opportunity for digital phenotyping to potentially enable closer monitoring of child and parental health.

Data collected by new digital devices opens an avenue for mining through artificial intelligence (AI) and predictive analytics, to convert real-world data into real-world evidence. Although there are challenges of telehealth and AI in medicine, the need to integrate health and health care systems into a cohesive ecostructure to enable health care providers to constantly adapt, respond, and learn from the health ecosystem and the current expectations from modern parents is evident.

This article focuses on applying real-world data and real-world evidence by the use of population health science in automated digital health and childhood obesity. It reviews current literature and shares practice evidence from Singapore, where the currently available technologies allowed the development of a digital televillage for child health. It describes experiences with the role of clinician in automated digital health, potential uses and abuses related to the implementations of automated digital health, and the assessment of outcomes of automated digital health in childhood obesity. The article concludes by describing what a digital learning health ecosystem for child health might look like.

TELEHEALTH, AUTOMATED DIGITAL HEALTH, AND THE INTERNET OF THINGS IN PEDIATRICS

Telehealth, including telecommunications and virtual technology, can help reshape and improve delivery of child health. The different domains of telehealth include tele-collaboration, teletreatment, telemonitoring, and telesupport, and the requisite standards are clearly defined by various governing authorities.[1–6]

The 'Internet-of-Things (IoT)", coined by Kevin Ashton in 1999, refers to a system of interrelated computing devices, mechanical and digital machines, objects, or people that are provided with unique identifiers and the ability to transfer data over a network without requiring human-to-human or human-to-computer interaction, bridging the health care environment and the community at large.[7]

The Digital Space for Personalized Child Health

Teleconsultations

Medical consultations have been enhanced through teleconsultations, both between providers and patients and between providers (**Fig. 1**). Such consultations can be used for follow-up clinical care or for new consultations. Health care providers play an important role in the appropriate selection of patients because not every type of patient can be managed through a teleconsultation. The role of teleconsultation will continue to grow as both evidence for and confidence in this modality develop and clinicians learn more about its potential pitfalls and challenges. In the United Kingdom, Babylon Health[8,9] has introduced such teleconsultations systems. At KK Women's & Children's Hospital in Singapore, we have set up the Smart Health Video Consultation Platform (**Box 1**) for teleconsultation. The system allows for scalability across the health care sector with economies of scale, and pilot data have shown time savings per session for the teleconsultations on this platform.

Medical devices and biosensors

Besides the digitalization of analog medical devices such as the stethoscope,[10,11] as well as the increasing use of transcutaneous bilirubinometers in the monitoring of jaundice in children,[12,13] the advent of wireless devices/biosensors, particularly those that

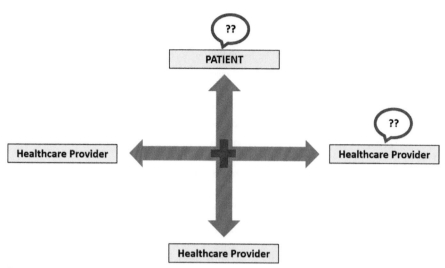

Fig. 1. Teleconsultations between health care providers/physicians and patients and between health care providers/physicians and health care providers/physicians.

monitor vital signs, electrocardiograms, glucose, and other point-of-care results, might play a pivotal role in child health in the coming years.

RAPID (Real-time Adaptive and Predictive Indicator of Deterioration) is a project from Birmingham Children's Hospital. This 3-year study funded by the UK Department of Health and the Wellcome Trust used real-time monitoring technology pioneered by McLaren from Formula One. Patch devices with wireless technology continually monitored data from patients, such as heart rate, breathing rate, and oxygen saturation.[14,15]

Biosensor wearables are becoming increasingly common and available. As consumer-grade devices such as Apple Watch and Fitbit continue to evolve with improved accuracy and integration with other digital devices and apps, many are looking toward the health care space to increase their market share. There is a growing opportunity for collaboration between the various stakeholders, such as the companies, engineers, and health care sectors, to develop clinical solutions for the assessment and treatment of patients. These wireless biosensors have a longer battery life, and many are water resistant and do not compromise patient comfort. They can monitor vital signs continually, upload the data into an analytical platform, and provide early-warning scores.[16,17] Virtual teleconsultations can be enhanced when biosensors provide real-time vital signs of the patient across the Internet to the health care provider. Algorithms can also be used to help the provider better understand the immediate care needed. In the community, patients can use these disposable wearables to monitor their medical conditions. In the future, it is reasonable to envision children with asthma putting on wearables and using predictive analytics connected to the cloud to review their real-time vital signs (ie, oxygen saturation and heart rate) and predict the severity of their asthmatic attacks, giving specific personalized and focused instructions on how to mitigate the asthma attack, including how many puffs of bronchodilators to administer and when to go to the nearest emergency department.

Social media, apps, chatbots, and digital phenotyping in child health

The health of children goes beyond the physical, mental, and psychological wellness of the individual and is connected with the community at large and influenced by

---

Box 1
Features of a smart health video consultation platform

Multiparty conferencing feature to facilitate a variety of health care programs and cross-institutional collaboration.

High video and audio quality and reliability, with reduced call drops over the Internet.

Leverage consumer mobile devices for ease of access.

Interoperability: caters for future integration with national health IT systems for seamless user experience.

Secure cloud-based platform: protected by proven technologies such as 2-factor authentication and end-to-end encryption.

Customer self-care portal that allows appointments to be made via e-mail and or SMS (short message service).

---

environmental, socioeconomic, and many other factors. The advent of the internet and cloud technology has created an interconnected and sharing community. It can be argued that the internet and social media represent the twenty-first century iteration of this ecological-environmental interconnected system. Clinicians should leverage on the social media platform as an opportunity to create a televillage to advance and improve child health. Social media are also important platforms for health care institutions and providers to provide credible and evidence-based information.

Apps can be used to help people with specific needs; for instance, children with special needs. The current cyberuniverse is rife with apps for children with these special needs.[18] It is thus important for these apps to be evaluated in a transparent and systematic manner so that health care providers are able to provide evidence-based advice for their patients.

A chatbot is a software with artificial intelligence (AI) that simulates a conversation/chat using natural language via messaging applications, Web sites, mobile apps, or through the telephone.[19] Chatbots may help in providing timely health advice for patients and families. They could address queries concerning specific diseases and escalate these queries to trained health care professionals when indicated. Caution is needed with such medical advice, and safeguards need to be put in place so that such advice is not misconstrued or misunderstood. Users should be given ways to connect with health care providers should they remain unsure of what to do after receiving such advice. Because it involves the general health and well-being (and morbidity) of children, implementation of such medical chatbots must be properly planned and evaluated before implementation. Similar to the health care apps, the postimplementation evaluation of medical chatbots should also be conducted.

A nudge, as defined by Thaler and Sunstein,[20–23] is "any aspect of the choice architecture that alters people's behavior in a predictable way without forbidding any options or significantly changing their economic incentives." There are health nudges now emerging to help drive proper child health behavior toward vaccination and healthy eating.[24,25] Moving forward, smart health nudges with robust design architecture with feedback loops and machine learning (ML) to improve the nudges and customize them to the individual needs of the population should be developed and are technically achievable at this stage of the digital revolution.

As described by Jukka-Pekka Onnela,[26–28] digital phenotyping is the "moment-by-moment quantification of the individual-level human phenotype in situ using data from personal digital devices" (in particular smartphones). Although still in development, digital phenotyping can potentially be used to identify postpartum depression or significant stress or depression in teenagers, through the digital signals they emanate. Increasingly, individual and population health behavioral preferences can be monitored and collected, and these repositories of behavioral health data can help clinicians as a community when they evaluate population health science and practices and develop new approaches to shape better health for children.

In short , the use of telehealth and telecommunications from teleconsultations, and the use of wireless biosensors, apps, and chatbots, although concurrently leveraging on social media to shape pediatric health behaviors, creates much opportunity for clinicians to improve health care and population health in pediatrics. Separately, these digital technologies have limited ability to effect change in child health but, if they are integrated together, they provide greater opportunities to enhance child health. The integration of digital technologies can be made possible only through collaborative efforts between various stakeholders on an individual and population level. Ultimately, a sustainable digital learning child health ecosystem can be built using AI and ML through real world data (RWD) and evidence to continually improve child health in this televillage (**Fig. 2**).

BIG DATA, ARTIFICIAL INTELLIGENCE, AND PREDICTIVE ANALYSIS: CONVERTING REAL-WORLD DATA TO REAL-WORLD EVIDENCE

In this fourth industrial revolution, data has been called the new oil[29] and AI the new electricity. There has been an exponential increase in data analytic advances in medicine over recent years,[30] and the potential of AI becomes increasingly evident.

In medicine, RWD are the data relating to patient health status and/or the delivery of health care routinely collected from a variety of sources. RWD can come from several sources and include electronic health records (EHRs); investigations from laboratory, radiology, electrocardiogram, and other point-of-care tests, genetics, and so forth); claims and billing activities; product and disease registries, patient-generated data, including in-home use settings; and data gathered from other sources that can inform on health status, such as mobile devices, including vital signs, point-of-care tests, and behavioral health patterns. Some RWD are complex and require data mining refinement before it can be used for further analysis and for translation into real-world evidence. EHRs, with their wide, disparate information, requires data mining. Health care providers, administrators, and technology providers should work closely together to ensure that the clinically important data can be easily mined and provide building blocks for development of evidence-based health care and the integration of AI.

Data will enable the development of an evidence-driven health care system.[30] Real-world evidence (RWE) is the clinical evidence regarding the usage and potential benefits or risks derived from analysis of RWD. RWE can be generated by different study designs or analyses, including, but not limited to, randomized trials, including large simple trials, pragmatic trials, and observational prospective and/or retrospective studies.[31]

AI is "a field of science and engineering concerned with the computational understanding of what is commonly called intelligent behavior, and with the creation of artefacts that exhibit such behavior."[32–42] ML, of which deep learning is a subset, was coined in 1959 by Arthur Samuel. ML is a critical component to AI development and finds patterns in data and then predicts the outcome (**Box 2**). In essence, AI and ML are the tools that are used to analyze RWD and develop RWE and translate these

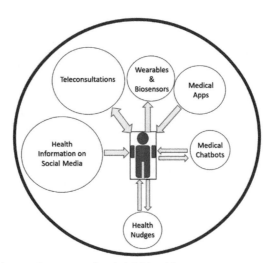

Fig. 2. The digital space for personalized child health.

into real-world algorithms for ultimate patient health care. An example of ML on the Web is Google's Deep Mind.

Kokol and colleagues[43] reviewed AI in pediatrics from a bibliometric perspective and, using a thematic analysis, identified 6 domains in the literature (**Table 1**). Through data-generated evidence, clinical decision-support systems (CDSSs) can be set up to improve health care delivery and health.[30] A CDDS is a health information technology system that is designed to provide physicians and other health professionals with clinical decision-making tasks. As Hayward and Neupert[30] from the Centre for Health Evidence put it: "CDDS link health observations with health knowledge to influence health choices by clinicians for improved health care." CDSSs constitute a major topic in AI in medicine.

Through ML, clinical algorithms can be set up to drive clinical decision making.[44–46] Increasingly, there are examples of this happening in clinical care. Specific pediatric examples include identifying children with autism, developing algorithms to manage pediatric sepsis, and developing a pediatric risk score that is integrated into the EHR and provides an early warning sign for clinical deterioration.[47–49]

Some RWD are complex and require data mining refinement before they can be used for further analysis and for translation into RWE. With its wide and disparate amount of information, EHR requires data mining.

Liang and colleagues[50] recently used ML classifiers to query EHRs in a manner similar to the hypothetical-deductive reasoning used by physicians and unearthed associations that previous statistical methods did not find. Their model applied an automated natural language processing system using deep learning techniques to extract clinically relevant information from EHRs. In total, 101.6 million data points from 1,362,559 pediatric patient visits presenting to a major referral center were analyzed to train and validate the framework. Their model showed high diagnostic accuracy across multiple organ systems and was comparable with experienced pediatricians in diagnosing common childhood diseases. It suggests that implementing an AI-based system as a means to aid physicians in tackling large amounts of data, augmenting diagnostic evaluations, and to provide clinical decision support in cases of diagnostic uncertainty or complexity is possible in the near future.

Box 2
Machine learning: types, models, and classification algorithms

Some common types of learning algorithms:
- Supervised learning.
- Unsupervised learning.
- Reinforcement learning.
- Feature learning.
- Sparse dictionary learning.
- Anomaly detection and association rules.
- Deep learning (or deep structured learning or hierarchical learning) is a type of ML that requires computer systems to iteratively perform calculations to determine patterns by itself based on artificial neural networks. Deep learning is essentially an autonomous, self-teaching system in which existing data are used to train algorithms to find patterns and then use that knowledge to make predictions about new data.

Various models used in performing ML (which is trained on some training data and then can process additional data to make predictions)
- Artificial neural networks
- Decision trees
- Support vector machines
- Bayesian networks
- Genetic algorithms

Types of classification algorithms in ML:
- Linear classifiers: logistic regression, naive Bayes classifier
- Nearest neighbor
- Support vector machines
- Decision trees
- Boosted trees
- Random forest
- Neural networks

Data from Refs.[35,39–41]

Challenges of Telehealth and Artificial Intelligence in Medicine

Although certain benefits are obvious, there are several challenges related to the application of telehealth and AI in pediatric medicine.

First, the sustainability of AI and the need for continuing AI learning has been recognized as a challenge. The Google Flu Trend was very promising when it was first launched in 2013 but the algorithm lost its accuracy as time wore on,[51] which shows that, although big data can play a substantial and impactful role in clinical care, clinicians must also be aware of their limitations and the potential hubris of any big data applications.[52–54] There is the need for continuous ML, akin to continuing medical education for pediatricians when new information and data are uploaded and refreshed on the existing models and algorithms set down. The IBM Watson tool was similarly touted to be the AI for new medicine but now its role has been questioned.

Second, AI and deep learning are often ultimately a "black box." Although human beings accept the heuristics of their decision making, as AI in medicine becomes more complex, there are increasing concerns about the black box of AI or of deep learning.[55] Human beings can only process so much data and, as they try to process massive amounts of data, the relative human-to-machine decision-making effort shifts to ML. This process creates a black box in the understanding of how AI arrives at complex decisions. This outcome has also legal implications: although there are existing standards set down by the Health Insurance Portability and Accountability Act (HIPAA)

Table 1
Artificial intelligence in pediatrics: a bibliometric perspective

Theme	Applications
AI in brain mapping	Prediction of child brain maturity, brain functional connectivity in preterm infants, classifying individuals at high risk for psychosis/pediatric unipolar depression/analysis of resting-state brain function for attention-deficit/hyperactivity disorder, predicting the language outcomes following cochlear implantation and so forth
AI use in pattern recognition	Seizure prediction in children with epilepsy; visualization of complex data[20]; predicting neurodevelopment; identifying motor abnormalities; analyzing EMG, ECG, and other signals; image analysis; segmentation; and so forth
AI use in pediatric oncology and gene profiling	Identification of regenerating bone marrow cell populations, benchmarking key genes for cancer drug development, gene expression profiling for children with neuroblastoma or lymphoblastic leukemia
AI use in developmental disorders	Quantifying risk for anxiety disorders in preschool children, developing socially intelligent robots as possible educational or therapeutic toys for children with autism, identifying children with autism based on face abnormality and so forth
AI in pediatric emergency care	Automated appendicitis risk stratification, supporting diagnostic decisions, traumatic brain injury, and detection of low-volume blood loss
ML approaches	Artificial neural networks, support vector machines, decision trees and bayesian networks

Abbreviation: EMG, electromyogram.
Data from Kokol P, Završnik J, Vošner HB. Artificial intelligence and pediatrics: A synthetic mini review. Pediatr Dimensions, 2017;2(4): 1–5.

for compliance, there are still many legal issues that need to be sorted out in this new digital frontier, especially in health data protection and security.

With regard to its infrastructure, there is much cost that needs to be invested in setting up the ongoing infrastructural needs of a digital system, related to privacy and data protection issues. The interconnectedness of the global community raises risk issues concerning personal health data security and protection, particularly if it involves sensitive health data of patients. Systems must be put in place to properly secure and protect these databases.

Recently, federated learning[56–58] has been touted as a possible solution to guard privacy and yet increase the power of AI in medicine. Computing in a smartphone is now very powerful. This power will allow dissemination learning to be done off site on handphones in a distributed but connected, integrated, and safe manner.

Federated learning is a distributed ML approach that might minimize the risks of data security and ensure data protection.

APPLYING REAL-WORLD DATA AND REAL-WORLD EVIDENCE: POPULATION HEALTH SCIENCE IN AUTOMATED DIGITAL HEALTH AND CHILDHOOD OBESITY

The health needs in pediatrics have evolved, and Palfrey and colleagues[59] identified these millennial morbidities in community pediatrics, including overweight and obesity, increasing mental health concerns, and technological influences on health.

Population health science is an emerging field in health science that takes an interdisciplinary approach to addressing problems of population health, taking into account the biological, social, and behavioral determinants of health. This approach integrates public health with social science and other disciplines, and places health as an important consideration in decisions made in all societal sectors. Such a multilevel and coordinated approach is best shown by childhood obesity, where there are marked disparities by race, socioeconomic status, neighborhood, and access to health care. A successful approach will need to take into consideration not just the biological nature of the disease but also the societal influence of policies, social environment, and physical environment to alter the physical activity and eating habits of the family and child. **Fig. 3** shows an adapted framework introduced by the US National Institutes of Health–supported Centers for Population Health and Health Disparities using childhood obesity as an example to show the proximal, intermediate, and distal factors affecting the disease.[60] A promising example will be the multilevel approach to childhood obesity in Cambridge,[61] an ethnically and socially diverse urban community, which has led to a reduction in prevalence of childhood obesity in the community. This massive collaborative effort took 7 years from formation to implementation, and sustainability and automated digital health may potentially hasten the process and allow rapid translation in more communities. Automated digital health can potentially be deployed in the various proximal, intermediate, and distal factors to affect health outcomes. Integrating a multilevel approach using automated digital health can potentially enhance population health and provide data for more proactive approaches to diseases requiring such an approach.

Role of Clinicians in Automated Digital Health

The Expert Committee on the Assessment, Prevention, and Treatment of Child and Adolescent Overweight and Obesity mentioned the role of the primary care provider in the office to diagnose and manage childhood obesity.[62] These recommendations also cite motivational interviewing as one of the behavioral strategies for physicians to assess the family's readiness for change. However, diagnosis is difficult to implement because of time constraints and the need to calculate body mass index (BMI) and plot on a gender-appropriate and age-appropriate chart. Primary care providers may not be trained in motivational interviewing and may lack confidence and time in providing feedback on a child's weight status. Primary physicians also do not have the time to do a nutritional and physical activity assessment and provide personalized feedback.

Traveras and colleagues[63] showed how a computerized, point-of-care decision alert helps alleviate the challenges discussed earlier and showed a reduction in BMI of study participants with childhood obesity. The pop-up alert includes several parts: (1) generate an automated alert on child's BMI percentile, (2) document a diagnosis of obesity, (3) discuss nutrition and physical activity, and (4) provide educational

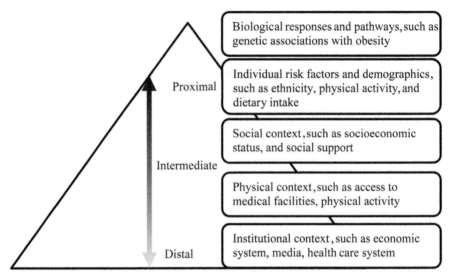

Fig. 3. Population health science model of childhood obesity that leads to disparate health outcomes.

materials. Follow-up phone coaching by health educators trained in motivational interviewing with automated text messages was also incorporated in the intervention.

With the advent of wearables, integrating tracking data with personalized feedback and prompts, as detailed earlier, is a potentially powerful tool to be used in the management of chronic diseases. Clinicians can still be an important resource in monitoring growth, providing evidence-based information, and troubleshooting in areas that families are struggling with.

Implementations of Automated Digital Health for Childhood Obesity: Its Potential Uses and Abuses

Some of the possible opportunities that automated digital health provides that are currently still under investigation include allowing the tracking of lifestyle changes; providing rapid real-time, personalized feedback and interactivity through data analytics and AI and reducing dropout rates; integrating data from wearables; and its accessibility, especially to the young.

However, with the widespread use of social media, adolescents are susceptible to cyberbullying and Internet addiction. Privacy issues are also areas that the laws struggle to catch up with internationally. With the sleep-wake cycle reversal common in adolescence, excessive social media can potentially aggravate sleep difficulties, which can lead to overweight. Clinicians will need to provide anticipatory guidance to parents to supervise their children's digital usage.

Assessing Outcomes of Automated Digital Health in Childhood Obesity

Because of differences in the types of outcome measured and how the outcomes are being measured, it is difficult to interpret the effectiveness of automated digital health. Current research is limited by standardized outcome measurements, which do not take into account the unique features of each patient.

Various policy makers, stakeholders, researchers, and clinicians need to work together to have common terminology in assessment of outcomes in childhood obesity interventions. Before accurate assessment of interventions can be performed, clinicians first need to rely on a comprehensive assessment of both the family and child with obesity. Childhood obesity is a chronic disease with medical and psychosocial complications, and assessment of just 1 parameter is insufficient. The Edmonton Obesity Staging System for Pediatrics (EOSS-P),[64] which is adapted from the adult-oriented EOSS, stratifies patients according to obesity-associated comorbidities and barriers to weight management. The EOSS-P is a potentially powerful, simple tool for assessing childhood obesity. There are 4 graded categories (0–3) within 4 main domains: metabolic, mechanical, mental health, and social milieu (the 4 Ms) to help inform physicians on a stage-based management plan. Although the EOSS-P is based on common clinical assessments that physicians perform, it will be time and resource intensive to assess the 4 domains. Automated digital health can potentially alleviate that through self-administered questionnaires and to provide the clinician with the summary of the risk category that the patient is in so that the clinician's consult can potentially be more targeted and effective.

At present, the success of childhood obesity intervention is commonly assessed using BMI z-score.[65] Other outcome measures that are commonly assessed include quality of life and cardiometabolic parameters.[66] There are several limitations to using these outcome measures. Opportunities may be missed in highlighting positive lifestyle changes that a child or family may have undertaken that may predate BMI changes.[67–71] Researchers and clinicians may be similarly discouraged because the improvement may be diluted by varying levels and domains that each child is affected by in the 4 Ms (metabolic, mechanical, mental health, and social milieu). Thus, a comprehensive, standardized, automated assessment of children with obesity can potentially provide opportunities to improve patient outcomes, experience, clinical effectiveness, and patient safety.

DEVELOPING A DIGITAL LEARNING HEALTH ECOSYSTEM FOR CHILD HEALTH

What might a digital learning health ecosystem look like? The US Institute of Medicine (now National Academy of Medicine) defines a learning health care system as one in which science, informatics, incentives, and culture are aligned for continuous improvement and innovation, with best practices seamlessly embedded in the delivery

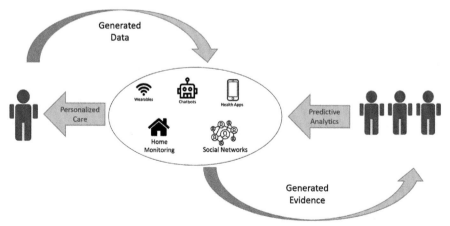

Fig. 4. Personalized care and predictive analytics for individuals and the population.

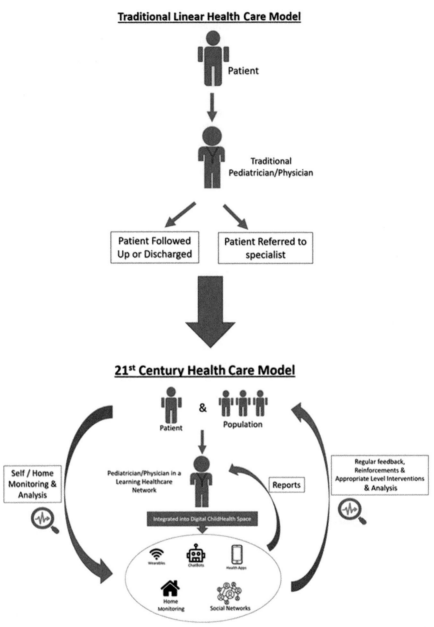

Fig. 5. The traditional linear health care model and the twenty-first century child health learning ecosystem.

process and new knowledge captured as an integral by-product of the delivery experience.

Science develops evidence that translates to care. Clinical care in turn provides RWD to develop new science, and the cycle continues. The televillage collectively involves clinicians, patients, and communities. Scientific data should be constantly

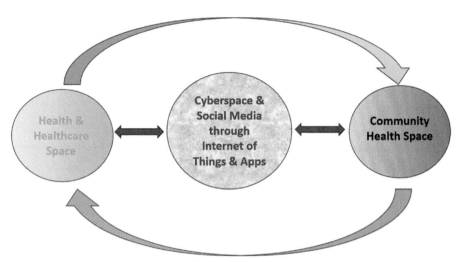

Fig. 6. Bridging the health/health care space and community health space with technology.

interrogated and translated back into practice on the ground. RWD and RWE should concurrently feed into this learning framework so that the ultimate result is an improvement in clinical care. Through technology and population study, predictive analysis can develop personalized care for individual patients. Data from individual patients will generate evidence and drive more population studies (**Fig. 4**).

The current health care system model is linear and, by design, wasteful, with little opportunity for learning and improving. This linear mode[68] is not set up to be a learning health care system, in which there are continuous loops of constant RWD and RWE with learning, reworking, and translation back into the real world and then back again. Technology can enable the development of a constantly learning health care system, with seamless integration of care to meet the core elements of a learning health ecosystem, transforming clinical care from the current wasteful linear model to one that is continuous and constantly learning and improving (**Fig. 5**). Technology will move the population health management from one that is hospital-centric to one that is village life–centric, where patients and population come in as active partners to cocreate value to this health ecosystem.[72]

SUMMARY

Reflecting on the evidence presented and our Singapore pediatric health experiences, it is necessary to move away from the traditional hospital-centric model of health care and instead take a life-course approach and use a life-centric model for pediatrics. Population health in pediatrics should be the overarching platform in pediatrics of the twenty-first century: clinicians should not just cure diseases but should improve overall child health. Health care efforts should complement and potentially enhance public health efforts, involving the various stakeholders, similar to the example of a multilevel approach to childhood obesity. Clinicians need to move upstream and address the health and not just the health care issues of children, and adopt proactive instead of reactive approaches as health care providers in pediatrics.

Technology and telehealth, if properly positioned, will improve the delivery of health to the population in a dynamic and responsive manner and can transform health delivery from the current largely reactive mode to a proactive one, especially when it comes to

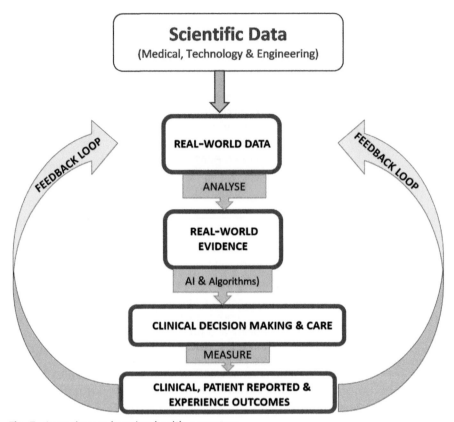

Fig. 7. A continuous learning health ecosystem.

promoting and improving health and not just managing diseases. Telehealth through social media cyberspace and IoT can bridge and provide solutions and interfaces between the current health and health care space and the community health space (**Fig. 6**).

Technology enables clinicians to capture big data and RWD in a continuous manner. AI and predictive analytics can help to make sense of RWD. Medical care can furthermore be personalized and calibrated to the specific and individual needs and requirements of specific patient sets and individuals. It enables clinicians to estimate the effects of targeted interventions on individuals and groups in diverse patient populations and translate these findings into impactful strategies to improve the overall health of children in the twenty-first century.

Clinicians can analyze and respond more promptly to various health and health care issues in pediatrics. Health care providers play an important role in providing anticipatory guidance, advocating for the evaluation of health care technologies, and creating an evidence-based platform for their communities. Technology calls for the collaboration of the various stakeholders to provide more integrated solutions, enabling clinicians to translate population science into population management. AI in pediatric, can enable a truly learning health ecosystem to be developed where RWD is continually leveraged to generate RWE to improve and enrich overall child health in the community (**Fig. 7**).

DISCLOSURE

The authors have nothing to disclose.

REFERENCES

1. Burke BL Jr, Hall RW. Telemedicine: pediatric applications. Pediatrics 2015; 136(1):e293–308.
2. About telemedicine. American Telemedicine Association. Available at: http://legacy.americantelemed.org/main/about/telehealth-faqs-. Accessed September 16, 2019.
3. Telehealth Programs. Available at: https://www.hrsa.gov/rural-health/telehealth/index.html. Accessed September 16, 2019.
4. What Is Telehealth?. Available at: https://catalyst.nejm.org/what-is-telehealth/. Accessed September 16, 2019.
5. Telehealth. Available at: https://www.who.int/sustainable-development/health-sector/strategies/telehealth/en/. Accessed September 16, 2019.
6. National Telemedicine Guidelines for Singapore. Available at: https://www.moh.gov.sg/docs/librariesprovider5/licensing-terms-and-conditions/national-telemedicine-guidelines-for-singapore-(dated-30-jan-2015).pdf. Accessed September 16, 2019.
7. Botelho B. IoT explained: What is the internet of things?. Available at: https://internetofthingsagenda.techtarget.com/feature/Explained-What-is-the-Internet-of-Things. Accessed September 16, 2019.
8. Babylon health. Available at: https://www.babylonhealth.com/. Accessed September 16, 2019.
9. Burgess M. The NHS is trialling an AI chatbot to answer your medical questions. Available at: https://www.wired.co.uk/article/babylon-nhs-chatbot-app. Accessed September 16, 2019.
10. Schuman AJ. Electronic stethoscopes: What's new for auscultation. Contemp Pediatr 2015;32(2):37–40.
11. Leng S, Ru San Tan RS, Chai KTC, et al. The electronic stethoscope. Biomed Eng Online 2015;14:66.
12. Okwundu CI, Uthman OA, Suresh G, et al. Transcutaneous bilirubinometry versus total serum bilirubin measurement for newborns. Cochrane Database Syst Rev 2017;(5):CD012660.
13. Maisels MJ. Transcutaneous bilirubin measurement: does it work in the real world? Pediatrics 2015;135:364.
14. Using F1 technology to transform healthcare. Available at: https://healthmedia.blog.gov.uk/2016/01/20/f1technology-transforming-health/. Accessed September 16, 2019.
15. Life-saving alarm system reaches 1,000 patients. Available at: https://www2.aston.ac.uk/news/releases/2017/march/life-saving-alarm-system-reaches-1000-patients. Accessed August 1, 2019.
16. Lambert V, Matthews A, MacDonell R, et al. Paediatric early warning systems for detecting and responding to clinical deterioration in children: a systematic review. BMJ Open 2017;7:e014497.
17. Matam BR, Duncan H, Lowe D. Machine learning based framework to predict cardiac arrests in a paediatric intensive care unit : Prediction of cardiac arrests. J Clin Monit Comput 2019;33(4):713–24.
18. Nations D. The Best iPad Apps for Autism Spectrum Disorder. Available at: https://www.lifewire.com/ipad-apps-for-autism-spectrum-disorder-4114202. Accessed August 1, 2019.

19. Chatbot. What is Chatbot? Why are Chatbots Important?. Available at: https://www.expertsystem.com/chatbot. Accessed August 1, 2019.
20. Marteau TM, Ogilvie D, Roland M, et al. Judging nudging: can nudging improve population health? BMJ 2011;342:d228.
21. Thaler R, Sunstein C. Nudge: improving decisions about health, wealth and happiness. New Haven: Yale University Press; 2008.
22. Thaler RH, Sunstein CR, Balz JP. Choice architecture. Available at: http://ssrn.com/abstract=1583509. Accessed August 1, 2019.
23. Navin MC. The ethics of vaccination nudges in pediatric practice. HEC Forum 2017;29(1):43–57.
24. Li M, Chapman GB. Nudge to health: harnessing decision research to promote health behavior. Soc Personal Psychol Compass 2013;7/3:187–98.
25. Cadario R, Chandon P. Which healthy eating nudges work best? A meta-analysis of field experiments. Marketing Science 2019. https://doi.org/10.1287/mksc.2018.1128. Published Online:19 Jul 2019.
26. Onnela JP, Rauch SL. Harnessing smartphone-based digital phenotyping to enhance behavioral and mental health. Neuropsychopharmacology 2016;41(7):1691–6.
27. Torous J, Kiang MV, Lorme J, et al. New tools for new research in psychiatry: a scalable and customizable platform to empower data driven smartphone research. JMIR Ment Health 2016;3(2):e16.
28. Brown K. Your phone knows how you feel. Harvard Public Health Magazine 2015. Available at: https://www.hsph.harvard.edu/magazine/magazine_article/your-phone-knows-how-you-feel/. Accessed September 22, 2019.
29. Garg V. Data is the new oil, AI is the new electricity, who is building the new railroads?. Available at: https://medium.com/@amitgarg/data-is-the-new-oil-ai-is-the-new-electricity-who-is-building-the-new-railroads-c8995faa8fd2. Accessed September 20, 2019.
30. Hayward R, Neupert PM, Institute of Medicine. Evidence-based medicine and the changing nature of health care: 2007 IOM annual meeting summary. Chapter 5: the promise of information technology. Washington, DC: The National Academies Press; 2008. https://doi.org/10.17226/12041.
31. Federal & Drug Administration. Real-world evidence. Available at: https://www.fda.gov/science-research/science-and-research-special-topics/real-world-evidence. Accessed September 16, 2019.
32. Ramesh AN, Kambhampati C, Monson JRT, et al. Artificial intelligence in medicine. Ann R Coll Surg Engl 2004;86:334–8.
33. Buch VH, Ahmed I, Maruthappu M. Debate & analysis - artificial intelligence in medicine: current trends and future possibilities. Br J Gen Pract 2018. https://doi.org/10.3399/bjgp18X695213.
34. Matthews I. What is machine learning vs deep learning vs reinforcement learning vs supervised learning?. Available at: https://www.urtech.ca/2017/01/what-is-machine-learning-vs-deep-learning-vs-reinforcement-learning-vs-supervised-learning/. Accessed September 21, 2019.
35. Marr B. What is the difference between artificial intelligence and machine learning?. Available at: https://www.forbes.com/sites/bernardmarr/2016/12/06/what-is-the-difference-between-artificial-intelligence-and-machine-learning/#b13c0e12742b. Accessed September 21, 2019.
36. Darcy AM, Louie AK, Roberts LW. Machine learning and the profession of medicine. JAMA 2016;315(6):551–2.

37. Koza JR, Bennett FH, Andre D, et al. Automated design of both the topology and sizing of analog electrical circuits using genetic programming. Artificial Intelligence in Design 1996;151–70. Available at: http://citeseerx.ist.psu.edu/viewdoc/download?doi=10.1.1.53.3544&rep=rep1&type=pdf. Accessed September 21 2019.
38. Beam AL, Kohane IS. Big data and machine learning in health care. JAMA 2018; 319(13):1317–8.
39. Asiri S. Machine learning classifiers. Available at: https://towardsdatascience.com/machine-learning-classifiers-a5cc4e1b0623. Accessed September 16, 2019.
40. Sidana M. Types of classification algorithms in Machine Learning. Available at: https://medium.com/@Mandysidana/machine-learning-types-of-classification-9497bd4f2e14. Accessed September 16, 2019.
41. Machine learning. Available at: https://en.wikipedia.org/wiki/Machine_learning. Accessed September 20, 2019.
42. Schuman AJ. AI in pediatrics: past, present, and future. Contemp Pediatr 2019; 36(5). Available at: https://www.contemporarypediatrics.com/pediatric-practice-improvement/ai-pediatrics-past-present-and-future. Accessed September 16, 2019.
43. Kokol P, Završnik J, Vošner HB. Artificial intelligence and pediatrics: A synthetic mini review. Pediatr Dimensions 2017;2(4):1–5. https://doi.org/10.15761/PD.1000155.
44. Lakhani P, Sundaram B. Deep learning at chest radiography: automated classification of pulmonary tuberculosis by using convolutional neural networks. Radiology 2017;284(2):574–82.
45. Povyakalo AA, Alberdi E, Strigini L, et al. How to discriminate between computer-aided and computer-hindered decisions: a case study in mammography. Med Decis Making 2013;33(1):98–107.
46. Tsai TL, Fridsma DB, Gatti G. Computer decision support as a source of interpretation error : the case of electrocardiograms. J Am Med Inform Assoc 2003;10(5): 478–83.
47. Crippa A, Salvatore C, Perego P, et al. Use of machine learning to identify children with autism and their motor abnormalities. J Autism Dev Disord 2015;45: 2146–56.
48. Spaeder MC, Moorman JR, Tran CA, et al. Predictive analytics in the pediatric intensive care unit for early identification of sepsis: capturing the context of age. Pediatr Res 2019. https://doi.org/10.1038/s41390-019-0518-1.
49. Suresh S. Big data and predictive analytics: applications in the care of children. Pediatr Clin North Am 2016;63(2):357–66.
50. Liang H, Tsui BY, Ni H, et al. Evaluation and accurate diagnoses of pediatric diseases using artificial intelligence. Nat Med 2019;25(3):433–8.
51. Lazer D, Kennedy R, King G, et al. Big Data. The parable of google flu: traps in big data analysis. Science 2014;343(6176):1203–5.
52. Cabitza F, Rasoini R, Gensini GF. Unintended consequences of machine learning in medicine. JAMA 2017;318(6):517–8.
53. Chen JH, Asch SM. Machine learning and prediction in medicine — beyond the peak of inflated expectations. N Engl J Med 2017;376(26):2507–9.
54. Hun-Sung Kim H-S, Kim JH. Proceed with caution when using real world data and real world evidence. J Korean Med Sci 2019;34(4):e28.
55. London AJ. Artificial intelligence and black-box medical decisions: accuracy versus explainability. Hastings Cent Rep 2019. https://doi.org/10.1002/hast.973.

56. Bonawitz K, Eichner H, Grieskamp W, et al. Towards federated learning at scale: system design. Proceedings of the 2nd SysML Conference, Palo Alto (CA), 22 March 2019. https://arxiv.org/pdf/1902.01046.pdf.

57. McMahan HB, Ramage D. Federated learning: Collaborative machine learning without centralized training data, April 2017. Available at: https://ai.googleblog.com/2017/04/federated-learning-collaborative.html. Accessed September 16, 2019.

58. Bhattacharya S. The New Dawn of AI: Federated Learning. Democratized and Personalized AI, with Privacy by Design. Available at: https://towardsdatascience.com/the-new-dawn-of-ai-federated-learning-8ccd9ed7fc3a. Accessed September 20, 2019.

59. Palfrey JS, Tonniges TF, Green M, et al. Introduction: Addressing the millennial morbidity :-the context of community pediatrics. Pediatrics 2005;115(4 Suppl):1121–3.

60. Warnecke RB, Oh A, Breen N, et al. Approaching health disparities from a population perspective: the National Institutes of Health Centers for Population Health and Health Disparities. Am J Public Health 2008;98(9):1608–15.

61. Chomitz VR, McGowan RJ, Wendel JM, et al. Healthy Living Cambridge Kids: a community-based participatory effort to promote healthy weight and fitness. Obesity (Silver Spring) 2010;18(Suppl 1):S45–53.

62. Barlow SE. Expert committee recommendations regarding the prevention, assessment, and treatment of child and adolescent overweight and obesity: summary report. Pediatrics 2007;120(Suppl 4):S164–92.

63. Taveras EM, Marshall R, Kleinman KP, et al. Comparative effectiveness of childhood obesity interventions in pediatric primary care: a cluster-randomized clinical trial. JAMA Pediatr 2015;169(6):535–42.

64. Hadjiyannakis S, Buchholz A, Chanoine J-P, et al. The Edmonton Obesity Staging System for Pediatrics: A proposed clinical staging system for paediatric obesity. Paediatr Child Health 2016;21(1):21–6.

65. Sim LA, Lebow J, Wang Z, et al. Brief Primary Care Obesity Interventions: A Meta-analysis. Pediatrics 2016;138(4) [pii:e20160149].

66. Ho M, Garnett SP, Baur L, et al. Effectiveness of lifestyle interventions in child obesity: systematic review with meta-analysis. Pediatrics 2012;130(6):e1647–71.

67. Armstrong SC, Skinner AC. Defining "Success" in Childhood Obesity Interventions in Primary Care. Pediatrics 2016;138(4) [pii:e20162497].

68. Milani RV, Lavie CJ. Health care 2020: reengineering health care delivery to combat chronic disease. Am J Med 2015;128(4):337–43.

69. Smith M, Sanders R, Stuckhardt L, McGinnis J.M. (Editors). Committee on the Learning Health Care System in A, Institute of M. Best Care at Lower Cost: The Path to Continuously Learning Health Care in America. Washington (DC): National Academies Press (US) Copyright 2013 by the National Academy of Sciences, 2013.

70. Olsen LA, Aisner D, McGinnis JM. (Editors). Institute of Medicine Roundtable on Evidence-Based Medicine, The National Academies Collection. The Learning Healthcare System: Workshop Summary 2007. National Academies Press (US) National Academy of Sciences, Washington (DC).

71. Foley T. The Potential of Learning Healthcare Systems. Available at: http://www.learninghealthcareproject.org/. Accessed September 16, 2019.

72. Maljanian R. Population Health Management –Toward a Life Centric Model with Consumer as Co-Creator of Value. 2018. Available at: https://populationhealthalliance.org/2018/05/27/first-blog-post/. Accessed September 16, 2019.

Workforce Shortage for Retinopathy of Prematurity Care and Emerging Role of Telehealth and Artificial Intelligence

Alejandra Barrero-Castillero, MD, MPH[a,b,]*, Brian K. Corwin, MD[c], Deborah K. VanderVeen, MD[d], Jason C. Wang, MD, PhD[e]

KEYWORDS

- Artificial intelligence • Neonatal intensive care unit • Premature infant
- Retinopathy of prematurity • Telemedicine • Very-low-birthweight

KEY POINTS

- Retinopathy of prematurity (ROP) is a retinal disorder that affects premature infants. With improved survival of preterm infants, more infants are at risk for ROP.
- Shortage of the ophthalmology workforce for ROP is a serious and growing concern.
- Image analysis using artificial intelligence algorithms combined with clinical information can predict ROP risks and has the potential to mitigate the widening gaps in ROP workforce.

INTRODUCTION

Retinopathy of prematurity (ROP) is a retinal vasoproliferative disorder that affects premature infants. Despite advances in technology and perinatal care for premature infants, ROP continues to be a leading cause of childhood blindness in very-low-birthweight (<1500 g), very preterm (28–32 weeks), and extremely preterm (<28 weeks) infants in high-income and middle-income countries, including the United States.[1–3]

[a] Division of Neonatology, Beth Israel Deaconess Medical Center, 330 Brookline Avenue, Rose Building Room 308, Boston, MA 02215, USA; [b] Division of Newborn Medicine, Boston Children's Hospital, Boston, MA, USA; [c] Department of Radiology, Cleveland Clinic Foundation, Imaging Institute, 9500 Euclid Avenue - L10, Cleveland, OH 44195, USA; [d] Department of Ophthalmology, Boston Children's Hospital, 300 Longwood Avenue, Fegan 4, Boston, MA 02115, USA; [e] Center for Policy, Outcomes, and Prevention, Stanford University School of Medicine, 117 Encina Commons, Stanford, CA 94305, USA
* Corresponding author. Division of Neonatology, Beth Israel Deaconess Medical Center, 330 Brookline Avenue, Rose Building Room 308, Boston, MA 02215.
E-mail address: abcastil@bidmc.harvard.edu

Pediatr Clin N Am 67 (2020) 725–733
https://doi.org/10.1016/j.pcl.2020.04.012
0031-3955/20/© 2020 Elsevier Inc. All rights reserved.

Data from the National Eye Institute report that approximately 1100 to 1500 infants develop ROP requiring medical treatment and approximately 400 to 600 infants in the United States become legally blind from ROP every year.[4] Annual expenses for visual impairment and blindness could be a significant economic burden, ranging from $12,175 (PPP adjusted) for moderate impairment to $24,180 for severe impairment.[5] More recently, there has been an increase in premature births as well as survival of periviable infants born between 22 weeks and 25 weeks[6]; consequently, more very-low-birthweight infants are at risk of developing ROP.[7] A recent cohort study from a large national pediatric database showed that there has been an increase in the incidence of ROP from 14.7% in 2000% to 19.9% in 2012, inversely associated with the decline in newborn mortality in the United States.[8] Concurrently, there has been a shortage over the past decade in the workforce of ophthalmologists caring for infants with ROP in the United States.[9,10] This imbalance between limited supply of ROP care providers and increased demand for services may put more infants at risk for ROP-related blindness and disability, which will severely limit their health, well-being, and educational potential in life.

RETINOPATHY OF PREMATURITY SCREENING CRITERIA

Currently, the official policy statement on screening for ROP from the American Academy of Pediatrics in conjunction with the American Academy of Ophthalmology, the American Association for Pediatric Ophthalmology and Strabismus, and the American Association of Certified Orthoptists (AACO), revised on December 2018,[11] proposes that infants with a birthweight of less than or equal to 1500 g or gestational age of less than or equal to 30 weeks, as well as infants with an unstable clinical course with a birthweight between 1500 g and 2000 g or a gestational age of greater than 30 weeks, should have retinal screening examinations until the retina is fully mature. In recent years, there also has been an attempt to reevaluate and more accurately identify infants at risk who qualify for ROP screening to potentially decrease the overall number of screening examinations by creating different prediction models.[12–14] These prediction models include additional factors associated with ROP beyond gestational age and birthweight, such as postnatal weight gain, as a proxy of the activity of insulin-like growth factor 1, and can be used as a predictor for ROP progression.[12–15]

CONCERNS ABOUT OPHTHALMOLOGIC WORKFORCE

Several efforts have assessed the workforce for ROP care, including workforce size, training background, and screening criteria. In 2009, Kemper and colleagues[9] identified ophthalmologists from an American Medical Association database and randomly called 9% (1504) of ophthalmologist offices to identify those who see children under 1 year of age. Completed surveys were obtained from 30% of ophthalmologists who reportedly see infants, and written surveys from these ophthalmologists were used to estimate that only 11% of all ophthalmologists screen or treat for ROP.[9] Ophthalmologists who provide eye care for children less than 1 year of age but do not provide care for ROP cited liability risk, lack of training or experience, screening for ROP being "too time consuming," insufficient reimbursement, perception of others providing the service locally, and cost of malpractice coverage as main drivers for lack of screening.[9,16,17] In a qualitative study of interviews with key ROP stakeholders (neonatal intensive care unit [NICU] and ophthalmologic providers) in 2 states, respondents perceived that legal liability and low reimbursement contributed to ROP provider shortages, supporting previous findings.[16] Additional surveys have further validated these findings and concerns about insufficient ROP workforce including a national survey of NICU medical directors in 2015.[18]

One of the major challenges related to the workforce for ROP care is that clinical ROP diagnosis is based solely on the appearance of retinal vessels on dilated ophthalmoscopic examination at the NICU bedside, which can be subjective and qualitative.[19] Previous guidelines recommended that examinations be performed by an ophthalmologist with knowledge and experience in order to accurately identify the location and sequential retinal changes of ROP through binocular indirect ophthalmoscopy (BIO).[1] Current American Academy of Pediatrics guidelines suggest that, if implemented properly, telemedicine systems using wide-angle retinal images and clinical data may be used for preliminary ROP screening or as an adjunct to BIO for ROP screening.

NATIONAL SURVEY OF RETINOPATHY OF PREMATURITY CARE PROVIDERS

Since the Kemper study in 2008,[9] we surveyed 500 pediatric ophthalmologist and retinal specialists who might provide ROP care, via purposive random sampling by 4 regions of the country in the United States. They were asked to anticipate practice plans for the next 5 years (starting from 2011). Ophthalmologist mailing lists were obtained from the American Association for Pediatric Ophthalmology and Strabismus and the American Association of Certified Orthoptists from 2011, and the survey was distributed and analyzed from 2011 to 2012, with a 62% survey response rate (previously unpublished [**Table 1**]). Of the 302 respondents, 64.9% (196) reported that they were currently providing care for ROP. Among those 196 providers, most were pediatric ophthalmologists (89%), but some were adult retina specialists

Table 1
Characteristics of retinopathy of prematurity care providers (pediatric ophthalmologist and retinal specialists) in the United States

Retinopathy of Prematurity Care Providers in the United States	N (%)[a,b]
Provides ROP care (n = 302)	196 (64)
Ophthalmology subspecialty	
Pediatric ophthalmologist	171 (89)
Retina specialist	21 (11)
Male	132 (67)
Area of practice	
Urban	120 (63)
Suburban	62 (32)
Rural	10 (5)
Midwest	45 (23)
West	46 (24)
Northeast	48 (25)
South	54 (28)
Setting of practice	
Private practice	113 (60)
Teaching hospital	71 (36)
Nonteaching hospital	7 (4)

[a] No significant difference between respondents and nonrespondents by region ($P = .36$).
[b] Not all ROP providers answered questions on sub specialty, gender, demographics, and practice.

(11%). A great majority of ROP providers (98%) performed screenings but only 54% performed treatments, consistent with data from Kemper and colleagues,[9,17] who reported that a smaller percent of ophthalmologists were treating ROP.[2] Additionally, we found that among the ophthalmologists who provided ROP care, 6.4% had no ROP screening examination training, 24.7% had no ROP treatment training, and 3.2% had no ROP follow-up training (examination after initial examination) during fellowship or residency.

In our survey, we found that, among ophthalmologists who were providing ROP care, approximately 15% did not plan to continue in the next 5 years (ie, by 2017), and an additional 4.5% planned to retire during the same period. Among the respondents, the authors found that there was a perception of shortages for (1) ROP screening examinations (48%), (2) treatment (45%), and (3) follow-up examinations (32%). Nearly all (93.3%) agreed that medical-legal liability for poor outcomes is a concern for providers, and 68.7% of providers disagreed with the statement, "compensation for ROP is adequate," consistent with previously published data.[9] These shortages likely will worsen over time unless innovative strategies are implemented, given the lack of interest in providing ROP care.[16] To counteract gaps in care coverage, the authors previously have suggested that coverage and reimbursement be linked to the full cycle of care for ROP, including screening, treatment, and follow-up in the first year of life.[16] This shift would require all institutions to ensure that preterm infants not only are screened on time but also that they undergo appropriate treatment and follow-up care prior to receiving full compensation.

POTENTIAL TO MATCH SUPPLY OF WORKFORCE WITH DEMAND FOR RETINOPATHY OF PREMATURITY CARE WITH TELEMEDICINE AND ARTIFICIAL INTELLIGENCE

Improved survival of premature infants combined with a relative shortage of ophthalmologists for ROP care has sparked interest in the use of telemedicine and artificial intelligence (AI) as potential solutions. Optical instruments for screening newborn retina have been used since the 1960s.[20,21] Traditionally, the gold standard for ROP screening has been the use of BIO.[11] Advanced technologies, however, including the use of wide-angle retinal imaging systems, have been used in the diagnosis of ROP for more than 20 years.[22,23] Although there are certain challenges with this technology, including image quality, variability of interpretation, equipment cost, and software compatibility with electronic medical record systems,[21,23–25] more recent studies have shown remote digital imaging to be a promising and cost-effective method of identifying infants who develop more severe ROP and potentially will need treatment.[26–28] These images can be taken by trained, nonphysician personnel and evaluated by a remote expert via telemedicine-based remote digital fundus imaging.[28–32] Multicenter studies comparing the accuracy and sensitivity of using BIO versus telemedicine showed similar sensitivity for zone disease, plus disease, and type 2 ROP, with a slightly better sensitivity with BIO for zone III and stage 3 ROP.[33,34] Currently, live ROP telemedicine initiatives successfully adopting the technology have been done in the United States, Germany, and India.[35–37] In the United States, the Stanford University Network for Diagnosis of Retinopathy of Prematurity followed premature infants eligible for ROP for 6 years, using remote retinal photographs by an ROP provider in 6 NICUs in California. During the duration of the program, telemedicine was found a safe, reliable, and cost-effective complement of ROP providers.[35]

AI and machine learning technology now are used in many areas of daily life to perform tasks or make data-driven decisions automatically.[38,39] More recently, this technology has been applied in health care settings in the form of complex networks of trained artificial neurons designed to create a model from data called deep learning.[40–42] Researchers in different areas of medicine, in particular, fields involving medical imaging, have studied deep learning technology and found it equal or sometimes even better in diagnosis than clinicians. In 2016, Gulshan and colleagues[43] developed an algorithm based on deep learning to detect referable diabetic retinopathy in adults, which has been validated in other countries, such as India.[44] A deep learning algorithm (i-ROP) also was evaluated for the diagnosis of ROP plus disease by testing the algorithm against 8 ophthalmologists, considered to be ROP experts given their clinical experience of more than 10 years and more than 5 peer-reviewed publications about ROP.[19] A convolutional neural network (CNN) (deep learning algorithm that assigns importance to different pieces of images to be able to be differentiated from one another[45]) was trained using a reference standard diagnosis as the gold standard. The reference standard diagnosis previously had been published as a reliable and accurate method of ROP diagnosis through a reference standard that puts together diagnostic information and a telemedicine system based on the image.[46] The sensitivity of diagnosing pre-plus disease or worse was 100% and specificity was 94%, outperforming 6 of 8 human experts.[19] More recently, the same group that developed the i-ROP developed a deep learning algorithm to track disease progression and regression after treatment and an automated fundus image quality assessment using a CNN can be done accurately compared with human experts.[47] These algorithms perhaps would provide clinicians with improved monitoring of ROP over time, even when patients are not located near an ROP center.[48,49] Other examples of this high performance in image recognition have been described in fields, such as dermatology, where neural networks were shown to classify images of skin cancer on par with dermatologists[50]; in radiology, to assess skeletal maturity on pediatric hand radiographs[51]; and in whole-slide pathology images.[52] Growing evidence has shown the ability of AI to bring specialty-level diagnosis to primary care settings; in 2018, the Food and Drug Administration approved the use of an AI-based device to detect some types of diabetic retinopathy.[53,54]

Added to the benefits of a comparable or even superior sensitivity or specificity to detect patterns compared with clinicians, computerized image analysis may offer a longitudinal view of serial images, learning from patterns, and gaining more insights in the progression of ROP and outcomes prediction. For example, a recent study has predicted cardiovascular risk factors from retinal fundus photographs via deep learning models.[55]

Although AI and related technologies still have limitations, understanding how deep learning analyzes data currently is an active area of research within the larger machine learning community. For ROP care, AI can be used to better stratify the risk profile of different patients and to match the risk profile of each patient to the limited supply of the ROP ophthalmologic workforce, in order to ensure more timely and targeted interventions. It also can mitigate the concerns for unforeseen ROP liability issues,[9] because every step of the care process would be documented with high degree of transparency,[56] with images captured, which can be used for research and teaching purposes.[57] **Table 2** describes potential benefits and barriers to the use of remote screening and AI models for ROP screening. Prediction models of infants at risk of ROP (discussed previously) should continue to be evaluated and validated in diverse populations in the United States and globally[12–15] as a way to lead to more-accurate screening and diagnosis.

It is possible that improvement in accuracy for screening will result in a reduction in the number of ROP examinations compared with the use of current screening guidelines. Finally, another positive benefit can be a decrease in unnecessary transports of

Table 2
Potential benefits and barriers of using remote screening using telemedicine and artificial intelligence for retinopathy of prematurity screening

Potential Benefits	Potential Barriers
• Image database may allow building more-accurate risk prediction models for ROP screening and progression • Use of images for research (clinical, outcomes, health services, and learning health systems) • Standardization of screening practices across diverse geographic areas • Images available for teaching purposes • Potential decrease in liability due to documentation transparency • Fewer transfers of at-risk infants to other institutions for ROP screening	• Change of NICU workflow • Change in clinical routines for ophthalmologists, which may lead to uncertain willingness to participate in telemedicine • Adoption of new technology will require staff training • Initial increased expenses related to new technology purchase and maintenance (cameras, computers, and software) • Training of technicians for telemedicine • Task shifting by telemedicine and AI may decrease the ability to maintain bedside skills of ROP care providers.

infants with multiple comorbidities associated with extreme prematurity who need to be transferred from one institution to another, where ophthalmologists can screen for ROP, although transfer still may be required for vision-threatening ROP and ROP treatment.[18,29] The need for bedside examinations and second opinions could be solved remotely through imaging analysis, improving outcomes and reducing costs.

SUMMARY

Timely ROP detection continues to be a concern, and, with improved survival, more infants are at risk of ROP. The worsening imbalance in the supply of clinicians and demand for services can be mitigated with more-accurate prediction models of who is at risk as well as through implementation of telemedicine and AI, including machine learning and deep neural networks. To accomplish this, the NICUs of the future will have to learn how to integrate technology into their workflow and care process that will include humans, machines, and evolving algorithms.

ACKNOWLEDGMENTS

The authors acknowledge the contributions of Monika Thomas-Uribe, MD, MPH; John A. F. Zupancic, ScD, MD (Beth Israel Medical Center, Department of Neonatology); Kristyn S. Beam, MD (Boston Children's Hospital, Newborn Medicine Department); and Andrew L. Beam, PhD (Department of Epidemiology, Harvard T.H. Chan School of Public Health). The research reported in this publication was supported by the National Eye Institute of the National Institutes of Health under award number 1K23EY018668.

DISCLOSURE

The authors have nothing to disclose.

REFERENCES

1. Fierson WM. Screening examination of premature infants for retinopathy of prematurity. Pediatrics 2013;131(1):189–95.

2. Spencer R. Long-term visual outcomes in extremely low-birth-weight children. Trans Am Ophthalmol Soc 2006;104:493–516.

3. O'Connor AR, Stephenson T, Johnson A, et al. Long-term ophthalmic outcome of low birth weight children with and without retinopathy of prematurity. Pediatrics 2002;109(1):12–8.

4. The National Eye Institute (NEI). Facts about retinopathy of prematurity (ROP). 2014. Available at: https://www.nei.nih.gov/health/rop/rop. Accessed June 8, 2019.

5. Köberlein J, Beifus K, Schaffert C, et al. The economic burden of visual impairment and blindness: A systematic review. BMJ Open 2013;3:e003471.

6. Patel RM, Rysavy MA, Bell EF, et al. Survival of infants born at periviable gestational ages. Clin Perinatol 2017;44(2):287–303.

7. O'Connor AR, Spencer R, Birch EE. Predicting long-term visual outcome in children with birth weight under 1001 g. J AAPOS 2007;11(6):541–5.

8. Ludwig CA, Chen TA, Hernandez-Boussard T, et al. The epidemiology of retinopathy of prematurity in the united states. Ophthalmic Surg Lasers Imaging Retina 2017;48(7):553–62.

9. Kemper AR, Freedman SF, Wallace DK. Retinopathy of prematurity care: patterns of care and workforce analysis. J AAPOS 2008;12(4):344–8.

10. Altersitz K, Piechocki M. Survey: Physicians being driven away from ROP treatment. Oculular Surgery News U.S. Edition 2006. Available at: https://www.healio.com/ophthalmology/retina-vitreous/news/print/ocular-surgery-news/%7Bedfa784c-a2ac-4f93-b473-5be5d07d82ca%7D/survey-physicians-being-driven-away-from-rop-treatment. Accessed July 1, 2019.

11. Fierson WM. Screening examination of premature infants for retinopathy of prematurity. Pediatrics 2018;142(6):e20183061.

12. Wu C, Löfqvist C, Smith LEH, et al. Importance of early postnatal weight gain for normal retinal angiogenesis in very preterm infants: A multicenter study analyzing weight velocity deviations for the prediction of retinopathy of prematurity. Arch Ophthalmol 2012;130(8):992–9.

13. Binenbaum G, Ying GS, Quinn GE, et al. The CHOP postnatal weight gain, birth weight, and gestational age retinopathy of prematurity risk model. Arch Ophthalmol 2012;130(12):1560–5.

14. Binenbaum G, Ying G, Quinn GE, et al. A clinical prediction model to stratify retinopathy of prematurity risk using postnatal weight gain. Pediatrics 2011;127(3):e607–14.

15. Hellstrom A, Hard A-L, Engstrom E, et al. Early weight gain predicts retinopathy in preterm infants: New, simple, efficient approach to screening. Pediatrics 2009;123(4):e638–45.

16. Wang CJ, Little A a, Kamholz K, et al. Improving preterm ophthalmologic care in the era of accountable care organizations. Arch Ophthalmol 2012;130(11):1433–40.

17. Kemper AR, Wallace DK. Neonatologists' practices and experiences in arranging retinopathy of prematurity screening services. Pediatrics 2007;120(3):527–31.

18. Vartanian RJ, Besirli CG, Barks JD, et al. Trends in the screening and treatment of retinopathy of prematurity. Pediatrics 2017;139(1):e20161978.

19. Brown JM, Campbell JP, Beers A, et al. Automated diagnosis of plus disease in retinopathy of prematurity using deep convolutional neural networks. JAMA Ophthalmol 2018;136(7):803–10.

20. Flynn JT, Cassady J, Essner D, et al. Fluorescein angiography in retrolental fibroplasia: Experience from 1969 - 1977. Ophthalmology 1979;86(10):1700–23.

21. Bulpitt CJ, Baum JD. Retinal photography in the Newborn. Arch Dis Child 1969; 44(236):499–503.
22. Chiang MF. Retinopathy of prematurity: Imaging in retinopathy of prematurity: where are we, and where are we going? J AAPOS 2016;20(6):474–6.
23. Valikodath N, Cole E, Chiang MF, et al. Imaging in retinopathy of prematurity. Asia Pac J Ophthalmol (Phila) 2019;8(2):178–86.
24. Wu C, Petersen RA, VanderVeen DK. RetCam imaging for retinopathy of prematurity screening. J AAPOS 2006;10(2):107–11.
25. Wallace DK, Quinn GE, Freedman SF, et al. Agreement among pediatric ophthalmologists in diagnosing plus and pre-plus disease in retinopathy of prematurity. J AAPOS 2008;12(4):352–6.
26. Chiang MF, Keenan JD, Starren J, et al. Accuracy and reliability of remote retinopathy of prematurity diagnosis. Arch Ophthalmol 2006;124(3):322–7.
27. Chiang MF, Jiang L, Gelman R, et al. Interexpert agreement of plus disease diagnosis in retinopathy of prematurity. Arch Ophthalmol 2007;125(7):875–80.
28. Salcone EM, Johnston S, Vanderveen D. Review of the use of digital imaging in retinopathy of prematurity screening. Semin Ophthalmol 2010;25(5–6):214–7.
29. Fierson WM, Capone A. Telemedicine for evaluation of retinopathy of prematurity. Pediatrics 2015;135(1):e238–54.
30. Mukherjee AN, Watts P, Al-Madfai H, et al. Impact of retinopathy of prematurity screening examination on cardiorespiratory indices. A comparison of indirect ophthalmoscopy and Retcam Imaging. Ophthalmology 2006;113(9):1547–52.
31. Yen KG, Hess D, Burke B, et al. Telephotoscreening to detect retinopathy of prematurity: preliminary study of the optimum time to employ digital fundus camera imaging to detect ROP. J AAPOS 2002;6(2):64–70.
32. Chiang MF, Starren J, Du YE, et al. Remote image based retinopathy of prematurity diagnosis: A receiver operating characteristic analysis of accuracy. Br J Ophthalmol 2006;90(10):1292–6.
33. Chiang MF, Melia M, Buffenn AN, et al. Detection of clinically significant retinopathy of prematurity using wide-angle digital retinal photography: A report by the American Academy of Ophthalmology. Ophthalmology 2012;119(6):1272–80.
34. Biten H, Redd TK, Moleta C, et al. Diagnostic accuracy of ophthalmoscopy vs telemedicine in examinations for retinopathy of prematurity. JAMA Ophthalmol 2018;136(1).
35. Wang SK, Callaway NF, Wallenstein MB, et al. SUNDROP: Six years of screening for retinopathy of prematurity with telemedicine. Can J Ophthalmol 2015;50(2): 101–6.
36. Lorenz B, Spasovska K, Elflein H, et al. Wide-field digital imaging based telemedicine for screening for acute retinopathy of prematurity (ROP). Six-year results of a multicentre field study. Graefes Arch Clin Exp Ophthalmol 2009;247(9): 1251–62.
37. Vinekar A, Jayadev C, Mangalesh S, et al. Role of tele-medicine in retinopathy of prematurity screening in rural outreach centers in India - a report of 20,214 imaging sessions in the KIDROP program. Semin Fetal Neonatal Med 2015;20(5): 335–45.
38. Beam AL, Kohane IS. Big data and machine learning in health care. JAMA 2018; 319(13):1317–8.
39. Hinton G. Deep learning—a technology with the potential to transform health care. JAMA 2018;320(11):1101–2.
40. Beam AL, Kohane IS. Translating artificial intelligence into clinical care. JAMA 2016;316(22):2368–9.

41. Yu KH, Beam AL, Kohane IS. Artificial intelligence in healthcare. Nat Biomed Eng 2018;2(10):719–31.
42. Jiang F, Jiang Y, Zhi H, et al. Artificial intelligence in healthcare: Past, present and future. Stroke Vasc Neurol 2017;2(4):230–43.
43. Gulshan V, Peng L, Coram M, et al. Development and validation of a deep learning algorithm for detection of diabetic retinopathy in retinal fundus photographs. JAMA 2016;316(22):2402–10.
44. Gulshan V, Rajan RP, Widner K, et al. Performance of a deep-learning algorithm vs manual grading for detecting diabetic retinopathy in indiaperformance of a deep-learning algorithm vs manual grading for detecting diabetic retinopathy in indiaperformance of a deep-learning algorithm vs manual. JAMA Ophthalmol 2019. https://doi.org/10.1001/jamaophthalmol.2019.2004.
45. Saha S. A comprehensive guide to convolutional neural networks — the ELI5 way. Towards data science 2018. Available at: https://towardsdatascience.com/a-comprehensive-guide-to-convolutional-neural-networks-the-eli5-way-3bd2b11 64a53. Accessed July 19, 2019.
46. Ryan MC, Ostmo S, Jonas K, et al. Development and evaluation of reference standards for image-based telemedicine diagnosis and clinical research studies in ophthalmology. AMIA Annu Symp Proc 2014;14(2014):1902–10.
47. Coyner AS, Swan R, Campbell JP, et al. Automated fundus image quality assessment in retinopathy of prematurity using deep convolutional neural networks. Ophthalmol Retina 2019;3(5):444–50.
48. Taylor S, Brown JM, Gupta K, et al. Monitoring disease progression with a quantitative severity scale for retinopathy of prematurity using deep learning. JAMA Ophthalmol 2019. https://doi.org/10.1001/jamaophthalmol.2019.2433.
49. Gupta K, Campbell JP, Taylor S, et al. A quantitative severity scale for retinopathy of prematurity using deep learning to monitor disease regression after treatment. JAMA Ophthalmol 2019. https://doi.org/10.1001/jamaophthalmol.2019.2442.
50. Esteva A, Kuprel B, Novoa RA, et al. Dermatologist-level classification of skin cancer with deep neural networks. Nature 2017;542(7639):115–8.
51. Larson DB, Chen MC, Lungren MP, et al. Performance of a deep-learning neural network model in assessing skeletal maturity on pediatric hand radiographs. Radiology 2018;287(1):313–22.
52. Bejnordi BE, Veta M, Van Diest PJ, et al. Diagnostic assessment of deep learning algorithms for detection of lymph node metastases in women with breast cancer. JAMA 2017;318(22):2199–210.
53. FDA permits marketing of artificial intelligence-based device to detect certain diabetes-related eye problems. FDA News Release. Available at: https://www.fda.gov/news-events/press-announcements/fda-permits-marketing-artificial-intelligence-based-device-detect-certain-diabetes-related-eye. Accessed July 19, 2019.
54. Abràmoff MD, Lavin PT, Birch M, et al. Pivotal trial of an autonomous AI-based diagnostic system for detection of diabetic retinopathy in primary care offices. NPJ Digit Med 2018;1:39.
55. Poplin R, Varadarajan AV, Blumer K, et al. Prediction of cardiovascular risk factors from retinal fundus photographs via deep learning. Nat Biomed Eng 2018;2(3):158–64.
56. Moshfeghi DM. Top five legal pitfalls in retinopathy of prematurity. Curr Opin Ophthalmol 2018;2(3):158–64.
57. Kemp PS, Vanderveen DK. Computer-assisted digital image analysis of plus disease in retinopathy of prematurity. Semin Ophthalmol 2016;31(1–2):159–62.

Competency-Based Training for Entrustment in Telehealth Consultations

Elaine Lum, MClinPharm, PhD[a,b,*], Louise Sandra van Galen, MD, PhD[c],
Josip Car, MD, PhD[d]

KEYWORDS

- Telehealth • Telemedicine • Telephone consultation • Virtual consultation
- Competency • Assessment • Entrustable professional activities • Medical education

KEY POINTS

- Telehealth consultations require the same degree of thoroughness and careful clinical judgment as face-to-face consultations.
- The distinct differences of telehealth consultations as compared with face-to-face consultations, warrant training in telehealth to ensure they are high quality, safe, and effective.
- Telehealth is now common and training should be incorporated into core curricula of medical schools and continuing medical education.
- Competency in telehealth consultations is suitable for operationalization as an entrustable professional activity.

INTRODUCTION

Telehealth can address approximately one-third (417 million) of the 1.25 billion ambulatory care visits and 34 million health visits in the United States annually.[1] Currently, telehealth penetration is low at less than 0.5% (1.25 million of 417 million potential virtual visits),[1] and sorely underused.

Telehealth consultations have been used for various purposes. For example, to triage and manage acute conditions, to support management of long-term illnesses

[a] Centre for Population Health Sciences, Lee Kong Chian School of Medicine, Nanyang Technological University, Level 18, Clinical Sciences Building, 11 Mandalay Road, Singapore 308232, Singapore; [b] School of Clinical Sciences, Faculty of Health, Queensland University of Technology, Australia; [c] Department of Internal Medicine, Amsterdam University Medical Center, Location VUmc, De Boelelaan 1117, Room ZH 4A58, 1081 HV Amsterdam, Netherlands; [d] Centre for Population Health Sciences, Lee Kong Chian School of Medicine, Nanyang Technological University, Level 18, Clinical Sciences Building, 11 Mandalay Road, Singapore 308232, Singapore
* Corresponding author. Health Services & Systems Research, Duke-NUS Medical School, 8 College Road, Singapore 169857, Singapore.
E-mail address: elaine_lum@duke-nus.edu.sg
Twitter: @ElaineLumx (E.L.); @GalenLouise (L.S.G.); @ejosipcar (J.C.)

Pediatr Clin N Am 67 (2020) 735–757
https://doi.org/10.1016/j.pcl.2020.04.013
0031-3955/20/© 2020 Elsevier Inc. All rights reserved.

pediatric.theclinics.com

(usually after at least one face-to-face consultation, although this paradigm is increasingly changing), to convey results of tests, for preventive health care (eg, reminders for vaccinations, uptake of screening programs, advice to patients in "teachable moments" during a telehealth consultation), and for home rehabilitation programs.[2–8] In pediatrics, telehealth services have included consultations in subspecialties; for example, burns, cardiology, child development, dermatology, endocrinology, gastroenterology, nephrology, neurology, oncology, orthopedics, surgery, and psychiatry,[9–11] as well as for speech-language services.[12]

Beneficiaries of telehealth range from patients to health systems.[13] Advantages of telehealth are related to service provision/accessibility to health care for geographically isolated patients (although there is evidence of high uptake in urban areas, bringing to the fore factors other than geographic distance); opportunity for greater relational/personal continuity (same clinician); complements or augments face-to-face clinic visits (follow-up care, earlier consultations when the patient is not as ill); potentially reduces waiting time for patients; minimizes travel either on the part of the patient/family or the clinician; reduces costs for patients and for service providers (although there is a scarcity of cost-effectiveness and health economics evaluation studies); and patient convenience (less disruption to daily routine, fewer days away from work or school).[9,13,14] Telehealth has also been shown to reduce environmental pollutants, minimizing greenhouse gas emissions caused by travel.[14] Challenges preventing widespread use of telehealth include issues related to reimbursement, as well as clinical (quality of doctor-patient relationship, quality of care), legal (licensing, credentialing, liability), and social (equity of access) concerns.[13]

The essential competencies required to practice medicine safely and effectively are equally applicable to telehealth. Telehealth consultations must be approached with the same degree of thoroughness and careful clinical judgment as face-to-face consultations. However, telehealth consultations differ in at least 2 aspects from face-to-face consultations: the absence of visual cues (telephone consultations), and not being able to personally conduct a physical examination of the patient (hence, losing therapeutic touch as a way to build trust and rapport, apart from informing the provisional diagnosis). In pediatric telehealth, these constraints are particularly challenging, as consultations with younger children are mediated via parents/caregivers more so than in face-to-face consultations. For example, in face-to-face consultations, the doctor may pat the child's shoulder (or another method of distraction) to reduce the child's discomfort during the physical examination, which is not easily replicated in remote consultations. However, similar to traditional consultations, the doctor would still engage directly with the child using age-appropriate language; for example, ask questions, clarify responses, and provide instructions. For older children and adolescents, the doctor may be able to engage directly with minimal or no mediation via a parent/caregiver. Especially for pediatric telehealth, doctors should be trained to be vigilant for clinical indicators warranting a switch to face-to-face consultation either in-clinic or making a home visit.

Good communication skills are foundational to the practice of medicine. Empathic and skillful communication contributes to building rapport, good doctor-patient relationships,[15] and patient safety,[16] whereas poor communication is a major source of patient dissatisfaction and motivates medical litigation.[17,18] For telehealth, highly attuned communication skills are critical for safe and effective consultations: skills in verbal communication, situational awareness, active listening, and insightful questioning are crucial, given the absence of many nonverbal cues, that is, loss of visual (telephone consultations), olfactory, and tactile cues. However, there is neither a consistent approach to teaching expanded communication skills for telehealth consultations,[19] nor is telehealth training embedded in medical school curricula.

We argue that training in telehealth consultations needs to be incorporated into core curricula of medical schools, specialist training, and in continuing medical education for 3 reasons. First, the sheer volume of clinic visits per year (up to one-third)[1] that can be delivered via telehealth, demand that telehealth training be part of core competencies. Second, the likely continued increase in telehealth consultations given its accelerated growth evidenced by a national study of US insurance claims in which usage increased by 53% from 2016 to 2017.[20] Third, that distinct differences in conducting high-quality, safe, and effective telehealth consultations as compared with in-person face-to-face consultations, warrant intentional training in distinct telehealth competencies (**Box 1**).

In this article, we do 2 things: describe the training program piloted with medical residents for entrustment of telehealth consultations, and propose telehealth consultation as an entrustable professional activity (EPA). Although telehealth encompasses a variety of synchronous and asynchronous modalities, this article focuses on a subset of telehealth: the provision of clinical consultations directly to patients via telephone and video consultations (**Table 1** shows differences between these and other telehealth modalities). Skills required by the patient/parent are not discussed, nor informed consent of the patient/parent for telehealth (eg, disclosure about advantages/disadvantages of telehealth, what they should be aware of before opting for telehealth);

Box 1
Considerations for telehealth (telephone and video) consultation training

Communication considerations for training in telehealth consultations include the following:
- Strategies to build rapport: use of minimal encouragers (eg, "uh-huh", "yup") to indicate attentive listening and acknowledge that the patient/parent is heard, tone of voice
- Telehealth etiquette: asking parent to switch to speakerphone (or video) mode if engaging with the child directly so they can listen in/be involved
- Use of plain language: avoid medical/technical jargon
- Check 2-sided comprehension: ask the patient/parent to summarize key points
- Invite the patient/parent to make notes and/or provide suitable education/information resources
- Recap key points and treatment plan at the end of the consultation
- Provide explicit safety netting: ask the patient/parent to call back if he or she has any concerns or if the condition deteriorates or does not improve
- Create a "hand on the doorknob" moment: let the patient/parent disconnect first to ensure he or she has no further issues to raise

Salient differences to face-to-face consultations for incorporation into telehealth training include the following:
- Setting up the consultation: ensuring a quiet environment, privacy, suitable and functional equipment
- Checking that the patient/parent is in a suitable/private environment and able to commence the consultation
- Beginning the consultation: self-introduction, verifying the patient's/parent's identity, and purpose of the consultation
- Guiding the patient/parent in self (child)-examination where appropriate
- Documentation of the consultation especially pertaining to signs and symptoms usually ascertained on physical examination. Patient/parent responses, expectations, concerns, emotions, comprehension; anticipated risks; treatment and follow-up plan should also be documented

Data from van Galen L, Car J. Telephone consultations. BMJ. 2018;360:k1047.

Table 1
Differences between telehealth modalities

Modalities	Synchronous	Asynchronous	Absence of Cues (V-Visual [ie, Able to See the Patient], A-Audio, T-Tactile, O-Olfactory)
Telephone	✔	✔ (voicemail)	V, T, O
Video	✔		T, O
Mobile messaging (text messages, instant messaging, messages within patient portals, in-app voice messages)	✔	✔	V (with the exception of sending photos/images), A (with the exception of in-app voice messages), T, O
Email		✔	V (with the exception of sending photos/images), A, T, O

neither are physician licensing, patient insurance coverage and billing, legislative limits of e-prescribing, and so forth.[21,22] The proposed EPA is a work-in-progress and we welcome further refinements and discussions. Definitions of key terms used in this article are provided in **Box 2**.

DEVELOPMENT OF COMPETENCY-BASED TELEHEALTH TRAINING

We developed a telehealth training program suitable for final-year medical students and medical residents, which could be adapted for established clinicians and other health professionals. Content of the training program was developed based on published literature on telephone consultations,[2,6,23–30] and present a strong foundation for expansion into specifics of training in video consultations.

Telehealth Training Program: Telephone Consultation

Learning objectives
Learning objectives for telehealth training comprising knowledge, skills, and attitudes (KSAs) were devised to encompass contextual background regarding telehealth, as well as to relate KSAs to various components of a telehealth consultation (**Table 2**). Learning objectives were mapped to the Accreditation Council for Graduate Medical Education (ACGME) and the CanMEDS competency frameworks (**Tables 3 and 4**).[31,32] Overall, the learning objectives (and hence, the EPA for telehealth) are underpinned by 2 additional elements: (1) trainees possess enabling or foundational clinical knowledge and skills for their area of practice; and (2) trainees possess global attributes, that is, the ability and willingness to self-reflect on practice, seeking and acting on constructive feedback, and timely referral.

Training format and resources
A training manual for trainers and trainees was developed based on the learning objectives. The manual comprised contextual background for telehealth, rationale for the training, learning objectives, training schedule and outline, and proposed assessment of explicit actions observed for telephone consultations. Training was provided face-to-face as a half-day workshop (5–6 hours including a 30-minute tea break) facilitated by 1 to 2 trainers/medical educators. Facilities required for the workshop

---

Box 2
Definitions of key terms

Telehealth

The World Health Organization (WHO) defines telehealth as the delivery of health care outside of traditional health care facilities that involves the use of telecommunications and virtual technology.[44,45] Broadly, telehealth can encompass clinical communication via modalities such as mobile messaging, email, health apps, telephone consultation, and video consultation. **Table 1** lists the differences between various telehealth modalities for virtual consultations.

Entrustable professional activities

Entrustable professional activities (EPAs) are professional practice tasks or responsibilities entrusted by the medical supervisor to be performed unsupervised by the trainee once he or she is deemed competent (via assessment/observed proficiency on multiple occasions).[45] As such, EPAs are the means by which competency frameworks are translated into clinical practice, and signal what trainees can or cannot do safely.[33] EPAs should be discrete, observable, and measurable (both in process and outcome), and may operationalize 1 or more required competencies.[45] The supervisor's decision to entrust the trainee with unsupervised practice involves assessing not only the trainee's clinical skills and abilities, but also self-awareness of their own limitations.[45]

Entrustment decisions may be ad hoc or summative (formal assessment) in nature.[46] Five (general) levels of entrustment and supervision for a particular EPA have been proposed: Level 1, not yet entrusted, trainee may observe but not execute the clinical task even with direct supervision; Level 2, trusted to execute with direct, proactive supervision; Level 3, trusted to execute with reactive on-demand supervision; Level 4, trusted to execute EPA unsupervised; and Level 5, trusted to supervise others in performing this EPA.[45,46] These supervision scales have recently been refined and validated for common pediatric subspecialty EPAs.[47]

Trainee

We broadly defined trainee as the individual undergoing training in telehealth consultations. Hence, depending on the context in which the training is being offered, for example, as part of medical school curriculum, during medical residency, or as a continuing medical education module, trainees may be final year medical students, medical residents, or established clinicians.

Telehealth training also should be made available to other (nonmedical) health care professionals. Hence, trainees also may be social workers, pharmacists, nurses, and therapists who are part of the health care team.

---

included a room large enough to hold trainees and trainers for presentations and group discussions, audio-visual equipment, and stations for telephone consultation role plays.

The workshop comprised the following components:

- Structured discussion of trainees' experiences with telehealth (case discussions including barriers, challenges, possible solutions) and their perspectives on required competencies
- Listening to and providing feedback about a trigger prerecorded telehealth conversation to elicit important behaviors, effective and ineffective practices in telehealth, recognize how the absence of visual cues changes the clinical consultation, recognize (hidden) concerns, and evaluate the use of physical examination

Table 2
Learning objectives (knowledge, skills, and attitudes) for telehealth (telephone and video) consultation training

	Learning Objectives for Training in Telehealth Consultation[b]
Background to telehealth	**Knowledge** K1. Appreciate that telehealth consultations are part of medical practice. K2. List diverse uses of telehealth consultations in medical practice (current and future). K3. Understand the advantages/benefits of telehealth. K4. Recognize distinct challenges/barriers and potential solutions for telehealth. K5. Understand that telehealth consultations require different competencies. K6. Recognize that conducting good telehealth consultations is similar to practicing good medicine in other settings. K7. Follow the technological developments that change telehealth consultations or require additional learning. **Skills** S1. Identify own preferred mode of communication. S2. Reflect on personal comfort levels for different forms of remote communication. **Attitudes** A1. Demonstrate interest in improving competencies in practicing telehealth consultations.
Components of a telehealth consultation	
Preconsultation[a]: Preparing for and setting up the telehealth consultation	**Knowledge** K8. List important behaviors in telehealth consultation. K9. Identify effective and ineffective practices in telehealth consultation. K10. Know the strategies for ensuring a private and quiet environment for the telehealth consultation. K11. Know how to use telehealth equipment; for example, telephone, hands-free headset, volume adjustment, recording functions (it is increasingly becoming a norm to record all telehealth consultations), video-conferencing equipment. **Skills** S3. Apply all possibilities to maintain privacy of the telehealth consultation from the doctor's side and verify at the beginning of the consultation that this is ensured also on the patient's side. S4. Adapt the physical environment to make conversation comfortable (eg, where possible, reduce background noise) and have every possible supportive device nearby. S5. Identify the patient's preferred mode of communication (eg, telephone, video consultation) and explain at what point those would convert to face-to-face (eg, poor connectivity).
Beginning the consultation	**Skills** S6. Establish that the patient is able to commence the telehealth consultation, has privacy, and is in a suitable environment. S7. Establish whether the consultation will be recorded (either by the doctor or the patient). S8. Identify the patient's preference for mode of communication (ie, phone call or in-person) for discussions regarding diagnosis and decision-making. S9. Explore and acknowledge the patient's perspective of the current interaction. S10. Explore the range of home management strategies available (including self-monitoring).

(continued on next page)

Table 2
(continued)

	Learning Objectives for Training in Telehealth Consultation[b]
The consultation	Knowledge K12. List essential tasks/skills in medical practice: K12.1 Identify ways to build rapport with patients. K12.2 Obtain a good medical history (including eliciting hidden concerns). K12.3 Ability for clinical reasoning. K12.4 Explore management options (assess the need for in-person treatment). K12.5 Negotiate a plan with the patient. K12.6 Follow-up and safety netting. K12.7 Deal with patient's (parents') emotions and expectations. K12.8 Identify necessary elements of documenting telehealth consultations. K12.9 List reasons for documentation of telehealth consultations, including legal aspects and continuity of care. K13. Acknowledge that the absence of visual cues (for telephone consultation) and not being face-to-face with the patient, changes how some of these essential tasks/skills are performed. K14. Outline reasons for adapting communication style for different groups and environments. K15. Describe unproductive patterns of communication. K16. Identify skills required for conducting difficult remote conversations. K17. Consider how the patient's personal context affects his or her experience of telehealth consultations (eg, hearing, cognitive, or language concerns). K18. Recognize limitations of family members or relatives serving as interpreters. K19. Recognize and discuss legal requirements of telehealth consultations in health care. Skills S11. Demonstrate the following essential tasks/skills in medical practice: S11.1 Build rapport with patients without face-to-face capabilities in telephone consultation. S11.2 Obtain a comprehensive medical history. S11.3 Recognize cues of hidden concerns through the telephone (and video) consultation. S11.4 Sound clinical reasoning. S11.5 Explore management options (assesses the need for in-person treatment). S11.6 Discuss and agree jointly on a plan with the patient. S11.7 Clarify follow-up and safety netting. S11.8 Deal appropriately with patient's (parents') emotions and expectations. S11.9 Document telehealth consultations with (at least) the same level of detail as face-to-face consultations, taking into account legal aspects and continuity of care. Research shows that documentation of telehealth consultations in electronic health records is often shorter than face-to-face; however, they require the same attention to detail (if not greater) in documentation.

(*continued on next page*)

Table 2 (continued)	
	Learning Objectives for Training in Telehealth Consultation[b]
	S12. Demonstrate strategies to address the absence of nonverbal cues for telephone consultation (eg, eye contact, gestures, facial expressions, posture, and the ability to see how sick a patient is). S13. Evaluate the use of physical self-examination. S14. Guide patients to perform self-examination. S15. Establish patient's (parents') level of health literacy. S16. Demonstrate awareness of patient's (parents') capacity to receive information (eg, attentiveness, emotional state, privacy). S17. Adapt verbal communication style to patient needs and mode of communication. S18. Demonstrate a flexible approach by adapting communication according to unanticipated situations (eg, recognize when interaction/communication is failing and make adjustments to rectify). S19. Use professional language in all communications. S20. Demonstrate solution-focused strategies for dealing with conflicts and uncertainties during telehealth consultations (eg, emotions, errors: your own or others'). S21. Maintain clear and appropriate records (hardcopy or electronic) of remote clinical encounters and management plans. Attitudes A2. Demonstrate commitment to conducting telehealth consultations with the same level of thoroughness and careful judgment as in any other medical setting. A3. Recognize the importance of effective communication in producing a good clinical outcome.
Concluding the consultation	Skills S22. Recap key points of the telehealth consultation for the patient (parent) and checks 2-way comprehension by asking the patient (parent) to summarize key points. S23. Provide education and resource materials based on levels of patient (parent) literacy (eg, reading, comprehension). S24. Clarify contact arrangements with the patient (parent), for example, availability, what to do in case of an emergency, call back if any concerns, contact details. S25. Share information only with the patient's (parents') explicit consent (eg, with family, third parties). S26. Letting the patient disconnect first to ensure he or she has no further issues to raise. Attitudes A4. Recognize their own limitations when it comes to conflict or uncertainty in providing health care remotely (eg, when and where to seek help, when to switch to in-person treatment).
Postconsultation	Knowledge K20. Identify gaps in their own knowledge base important for management of telehealth consultations. Skills S27. Self-reflect on performance. S28. Identify areas for improvement for future telehealth consultations. S29. Ability to view the telehealth consultation from the patient's perspective (for trainees, role-playing as the doctor). S30. Understand the telehealth consultation from the patient's perspective (for trainees, role-playing as the patient).

(continued on next page)

Table 2
(continued)

Learning Objectives for Training in Telehealth Consultation[b]
Attitudes
A5. Receptive to constructive feedback on performance.
A6. Receptive to improve on skills.

[a] This component is not applicable to an unscheduled telehealth consultation (eg, patient calls the doctor without prior appointment).

[b] Prerequisites are that (1) trainees possess enabling or foundational clinical knowledge and skills for their area of practice, and (2) trainees possess global attributes, that is, the ability and willingness to self-reflect on practice, seeking and acting on constructive feedback, and timely referral.

- Role plays with constructive feedback using an observation checklist; **Table 5** shows 1 of the 9 clinical scenarios used; **Box 3** lists the 9 role play scenarios designed to cover a variety of situations; trainees practice information gathering, developing rapport, negotiation, provision of education, and guiding patients in self-examination/assessment
- Discussion regarding documentation of telehealth consultations, that is, what to document, reasons for documenting, including legal aspects and continuity of care
- Concluded with self-reflection, debriefing, and workshop feedback

Trainee feedback on the pilot workshop

Six medical residents participated in the pilot training workshop (May 2018). A survey completed by trainees at the end of the workshop found that the learning outcomes

Table 3
Learning objectives for attaining telehealth (telephone and video) consultation entrustable professional activity (EPA) mapped against the Accreditation Council for Graduate Medical Education (ACGME) core competencies

	Learning Objectives for Attaining Telehealth Consultation EPA[a]		
ACGME	**Knowledge**	**Skills**	**Attitudes**
Patient care	K1-8, K12.7, K13	S6, S8, S10, S11.4–11.8, S12–14, S20, S22–25	A2
Medical knowledge	K12.1–12.6	S11.4–11.5, S13–14	
Interpersonal and communication skills	K9-11, K12.5, K12.8, K12.9, K15–18	S7, S9, S11.1–11.3, S11.6–11.9, S12, S15–26	A2-3
Professionalism	K10, K12.5, K12.7, K14, K15–17	S1–5, S6, S8–10, S11.8, S13–14, S17, S19–20, S25	A2
Practice-based learning and improvement	K7, K20	S27–30	A1, A4–6
Systems-based practice	K19		A2, A6

[a] This EPA is underpinned by 2 other elements: (1) trainees possess enabling or foundational clinical knowledge and skills for their area of practice; and (2) trainees possess global attributes, that is, the ability and willingness to self-reflect on practice, seeking and acting on constructive feedback, and timely referral.

Data from Holmboe ES, Edgar L, Hamstra S. The milestones guidebook. USA: Accreditation Council for Graduate Medical Education; 2016; and Stanford Medicine - Graduate Medical Education. Core competencies: being a competent new practitioner. 2018. Available at: http://med.stanford.edu/gme/housestaff/all-topics/core_competencies.html#patient-care-(pc). Accessed 10 September 2019.

Table 4
Learning objectives for attaining telehealth (telephone and video) consultation entrustable professional activity (EPA) mapped against the CanMEDS competency framework

| CanMEDS | Learning Objectives for Attaining Telehealth Consultation EPA[a] | | |
	Knowledge	Skills	Attitudes
Medical expert	K1–20	S1–30	A1–6
Communicator	K8–11, K12.1–12.2, K12.5–12.9, K13–19	S3–10, S11.1–11.3, S11.5–11.9, S12, S16–26, S30	A2–4
Collaborator	K12.8–12.9, K19	S11.9, S21, S25	A4
Scholar		S1–2, S27–30	A1–6
Leader	K1–5	S27–28	A1–3
Health advocate	K1–6		A2
Professional	K6–9	S3–30	A1–6

[a] This EPA is underpinned by 2 other elements: (1) trainees possess enabling or foundational clinical knowledge and skills for their area of practice; and (2) trainees possess global attributes that is, the ability and willingness to self-reflect on practice, seeking and acting on constructive feedback, and timely referral.
Data from Royal College of Physicians and Surgeons of Canada. CanMEDS: Better standards, better physicians, better care. 2019. Available at: http://www.royalcollege.ca/rcsite/canmeds/canmeds-framework-e. Accessed 6 September 2019.

were clear, the training was perceived to make a difference to the way they will conduct future telephone consultations, a personal learning goal was achieved, and the cases used for role plays were representative of their practice. Trainees suggested that supervisors also should be trained in telephone consultations, and to include adverse events/errors in telehealth for the updated version of the workshop.

The following key learnings were reported by trainees:

- The importance of patient verification
- The importance of asking patients to repeat or summarize key information to ensure comprehension
- Obtainment of a comprehensive, yet targeted medical history over the phone (often not done in practice)
- Use of a headset to free up both hands during a consultation (ie, to allow concurrent use of a computer and making contemporaneous notes about the consultation in the electronic health record)
- The importance of having a low threshold for converting to a face-to-face consultation (particularly in the case of safety concerns, comprehension issues, language barriers, and frustrations with the call)

Adaptations for video consultations

There are additional considerations for training in video consultation skills, depending on whether these sessions are assisted or nonassisted, by which we mean both technical assistance (support staff sets up the appointment, equipment, and connects the patient; all the doctor has to do is turn up and start the telehealth clinic session), and clinical assistance (whether a health care professional, eg, a nurse on the patient's side assists in the session, ie, physical examination, administering tests, and so forth). Doctors may need training in the use of proprietary video consultation systems particular to the health system where they work.

Table 5
Example of a role play scenario used in the pilot workshop: follow-up after blood tests

Patient: Mary O'Connor, age 42	Physician Calls Patient
Time	Monday 4.30 PM
Setting	Follow-up after bloodwork
Medical history	2015 Hypertension
Medication	Enalapril 10 mg 1 tablet daily
	Hydrochlorothiazide 12.5 mg 1 tablet daily
Family history	Father died of stroke at age 60
Social situation	Lives alone, has a dog
Intoxicants	Smokes 10 cigarettes a day, for 10 y
	A few beers on the weekend
Allergies	None
Part of physician	You make a call to Mary O'Connor, a 42-year-old woman who had blood work done several days ago on her last visit with you. She is a smoker and has hypertension. Her laboratory tests were all normal except for her lipid profile, with a total cholesterol of 260 mg/dL, high-density lipoprotein 35 mg/dL, and low-density lipoprotein 170 mg/dL. You want to start her on a statin.
Part of patient	You smoke half a pack of cigarettes a day, and you have no interest in quitting. You have hypertension, and take Enalapril and Hydrochlorothiazide for it. You saw the doctor last week and had fasting blood work done. During this call your dog keeps walking through the room and you cannot seem to concentrate.
Chief complaints	None
Answer only if asked	You have seen the ads for some cholesterol-lowering medications and have heard that they can have serious side effects. You are very reluctant to take these medications. Your diet is fast-food cheeseburgers 2 or 3 times a week for lunch, eggs for breakfast almost every day.
Hidden concerns	Afraid of side effects.

Box 3
List of role play scenarios used in the pilot workshop for medical residents

1. Patient with diabetes calls doctor for an unplanned follow-up telephone consultation.

2. Doctor (nephrologist) calls patient for a regular follow-up.

3. Doctor calls patient to follow-up after blood tests show an abnormal lipid profile.

4. Patient calls rostered doctor on Sunday to request Oxycodone (you are not this patient's regular doctor).

5. Patient with severe chest pain calls you (doctor) during your evening shift (you are not this patient's regular doctor).

6. Doctor calls patient to discuss test results and treatment of a sexually transmitted disease (directed to voicemail).

7. Patient (hearing impairment) calls doctor with a question about how much medication to take (new medication).

8. Talking to someone who is not the patient (with the patient's permission).

9. Patient calls doctor (on-call oncologist) on Sunday about new skin lesions.

Sharma and colleagues[21] make the following additional points about training in video consultations:

- Use slower speech to ensure clear enunciation
- Make movement/gestures in full view of the camera (however, minimize these)
- Use slower movement/gestures to avoid blurring over video
- Use a neutral background and good lighting
- Fix camera position to show clinician's head and shoulders in the center of the frame and to facilitate clinician looking at the camera for "eye contact"
- Dress in solid colors for optimal projection
- Use screen share to show images/diagnostic findings to patients
- Manage group interactions (patient, family)
- Be aware of and be prepared to activate emergency and urgent care centers in the area

Adaptations for pediatric telehealth

Although we have included examples of how selected skills can be adapted for pediatric telehealth (see **Table 2**) and suggested some scenarios for role play (**Box 4**), the development of a training package for pediatric telehealth would require input from pediatric health care teams, for example, pediatricians, pediatric nurses, and so forth. To inform and frame the development of such a training package, the core pediatric team could discuss the types of clinical scenarios to include in telehealth consultations, elicit barriers and enablers for safe and effective pediatric telehealth, and

---

Box 4
Examples of role play scenarios for general pediatric telehealth training

1. Parent of child with type 1 diabetes calls doctor after adjustment of medications a week ago (unplanned telephone consultation).

2. Video consultation initiated by doctor for a 10-year-old child with asthma (regular follow-up).

3. Doctor calls parent of child to follow-up regarding eczema treatment plan (video consultation).

4. Parent rings rostered doctor on Saturday, child on oral antibiotic for an ear infection since yesterday; parent is concerned that the child is still having fever.

5. 16-year-old patient calls to find out test results of a sexually transmitted disease (you are not this patient's regular doctor).

6. Parent calls doctor regarding a rash on their child's legs.

7. Follow-up video consultation of a teenager (female) recently diagnosed with anxiety and depression accompanied by the patient's mother.

8. Follow-up telephone consultation of a 4-year-old child undergoing chemotherapy for leukemia, monitoring/management of side effects.

9. Doctor calls parent of child regarding outcome of test results (directed to voicemail).

The development of a training package for pediatric telehealth would require input from pediatric health care teams, for example, pediatricians, pediatric nurses, and so forth. To inform and frame the development of such a training package, the core pediatric team could discuss the types of clinical scenarios to include in telehealth consultations, elicit barriers and enablers for safe and effective pediatric telehealth, and highlight any areas of concern or potential risk.

highlight any areas of concern or potential risk. Where possible and appropriate, mitigation strategies should be incorporated into the training.

ENTRUSTABLE PROFESSIONAL ACTIVITY FOR TELEHEALTH (TELEPHONE/VIDEO) CONSULTATIONS

In the interest of patient safety, competency must be demonstrated before the clinician conducts telehealth consultations unsupervised. Hence, the privilege to conduct telehealth consultations warrants a "gate," operationalized as an EPA, similar to what has been proposed for conducting patient handovers and for prescribing.[33,34] The use of EPAs are increasingly familiar to doctors, with peak bodies such as The American Board of Pediatrics adopting EPAs for various clinical tasks[35,36] and for physician training.[37]

We developed an EPA for telehealth consultations (**Table 6**) based on the learning objectives of the workshop, and published examples such as EPAs for general pediatrics by The American Board of Pediatrics.[33,35] The proposed EPA is a work-in-progress and we welcome further refinements and discussions, including the sources of information for formative evaluation of progress and the basis for formal entrustment decisions.

An arbitrary number of consecutive observations (ie, 10) has been proposed to be conducted proficiently without error (commissions or omissions), comprising a mix of telephone and video consultations, covering a cross section of patient age groups and telehealth agendas pertinent to the trainee's area of practice. Questions remain as to whether (1) the trainee starts over (starting the count from 1 again) if a consultation for example, the eighth consultation was not deemed proficient or error-free, (2) the merits (or otherwise) of imposing a strict consecutive count of such consultations, (3) the frequency/number of proficient and error-free consultations required to be deemed competent, and (4) the period of time over which the summative assessment can be done (ie, 10 proficient and error-free telehealth consultations in 6 months, 12 months? What is realistic in terms of opportunity and variety of cases for the setting?). In addition, documentation of the telehealth consultation must be assessed and judged to be adequate.

We proposed summative observations and evaluation of documentation to be performed by a total of at least 2 supervisors/attending physicians (eg, 1 supervisor may evaluate 3 telehealth consultations, another may evaluate 7) using a structured observation tool. The observation tool can be adapted from the skills stated in the proposed EPA; an example is shown in **Table 7**.

Another consideration is whether there should be an expiry date of the summative entrustment decision. For example, if the trainee has not conducted telehealth consultations for a period of time (how long?), the entrustment decision expires and the individual should be supervised again.

Before attaining entrustment, trainees should be exposed to observing (well-conducted) telehealth consultations, conducting telehealth consultations under direct proactive supervision, and conducting telehealth consultations with on-demand supervision. Entrustment of telehealth consultation is estimated to occur at the end of the first year of residency training.

The EPA for telehealth consultations also can be used as a teaching tool for final year medical students as part of consultation skills training, to create awareness, and to introduce these competencies. During internships or site placements, medical students should be encouraged/invited to observe a (well-conducted) telehealth consultation. Student observation of such consultations should not be regarded as

Table 6 Proposed entrustable professional activity (EPA) for telehealth (telephone and video) consultation based on published examples	
EPA Title	**Telehealth (Telephone and Video) Consultation**
Description of the activity	In this EPA, telehealth consultations refer to telephone or video consultations conducted by the doctor with a patient (with/without parents, caregiver, and family present). Consultations can be initiated by either the doctor or patient via a booked appointment, or may be an unscheduled call (eg, initiated by the patient). Telehealth consultations can be used for various purposes. For example, to triage and manage acute conditions, to support management of long-term illnesses (usually after at least one face-to-face consultation), to convey results of tests (where appropriate to do so), for preventive health care (eg, reminders for vaccinations, uptake of screening programs, advice to patients in "teachable moments" during a telehealth consultation), and for home rehabilitation programs.[2–8]
Mapping to competency frameworks	Detailed mapping of telehealth training learning objectives (curricular components) to core competencies of the Accreditation Council for Graduate Medical Education (ACGME) and the CanMEDS framework are provided in **Tables 3** and **4**. The most relevant domains of the ACGME core competencies are Patient Care, Interpersonal and Communication Skills, and Professionalism. The most relevant domains of the CanMEDS framework are Medical Expert, Communicator, and Professional.
Required knowledge, skills, and attitudes (KSAs) needed to execute this EPA safely	**Table 2** details the KSAs for this EPA underpinned by 2 attributes: (1) trainees possess enabling or foundational clinical knowledge and skills for their area of practice, and (2) trainees possess global attributes, that is, the ability and willingness to self-reflect on practice, seeking and acting on constructive feedback, and timely referral. A global summary of required KSAs is as follows: Knowledge Trainees must understand the diverse uses of telehealth consultations in medical practice; know the advantages, the limitations (including having a low-threshold for reverting to in-person consultation either in clinic or via a home visit), and challenges of telehealth, and the solutions to these challenges; know what needs to be adjusted for a productive telehealth consultation (in terms of communication and clinical consultation); and recognize that conducting

(continued on next page)

Table 6
(continued)

EPA Title	Telehealth (Telephone and Video) Consultation
	good telehealth consultations is similar to practicing good medicine in other settings.
	Skills
	Key skills include the following. Appropriate set-up of teleconsultation for ease of communication and patient privacy. Highly attuned and clear communication skills with patients (parents and family members, where appropriate), especially in the absence of visual cues (telephone consultation) and not being in the same physical space (instructions to patients [parents] for self [child]-examination need to be clear). Trainees must demonstrate their ability to perform essential tasks/skills in medical practice expected of a typical clinical consultation via telehealth; and be able to discern when to convert to in-person consultation either in clinic or via a home visit. To conclude the telehealth consultation and to ensure the patient is clear on the treatment plan, trainees must recap key points of the telehealth consultation and check 2-way comprehension by asking the patient (parent) to summarize key points; provide relevant education/information; clarify contact arrangements; and document the consultation and treatment plan.
	Attitudes
	Trainees must show a commitment to conducting telehealth consultations with the same level of thoroughness and careful judgment as in any other medical setting; recognize the importance of effective communication skills for a productive telehealth consultation; recognize their own limitations and limitations of telehealth (knows when and where to seek help, when to switch to in-person consultation); receptive to constructive feedback on performance; and willing to improve on skills.
Sources of information to evaluate progress (formative)	Structured observations during supervised telehealth consultations using an observation and feedback tool (the learning objectives in **Table 2**, eg, skills, can be adapted into an observation tool). Timely formative feedback to be provided to trainee.
	Seek and discuss self-reflection from the trainee.
	Case-based discussions with the trainee.
	Formative evaluation of the corresponding documentation of the supervised telehealth consultations.
	Anticipatory guidance, for example, "what if" discussions with the trainee to explore ability to cope with challenging case situations.

(continued on next page)

Table 6 (continued)	
EPA Title	**Telehealth (Telephone and Video) Consultation**
Estimated stage of training when Level 4 (unsupervised practice) is reached	At the end of first year of residency training (postgraduate year 1).
Basis for formal entrustment decision	At least 10 consecutive telehealth consultations (telephone and/or video consultations, depending on the modality used by the health service) observed by at least 2 supervisors/attending physicians using a structured observation tool, covering a cross section of patient age groups and purpose/s of telehealth consultations with the trainee in the health provider role. All 10 telehealth consultations must be conducted proficiently and without errors (commissions or omissions). The observing supervisors/attending physicians must evaluate the documentation of these 10 consecutive telehealth consultations by the trainee, and the documentation judged to be adequate.

Data from ten Cate O, Young JQ. The patient handover as an entrustable professional activity: adding meaning in teaching and practice. BMJ Qual Saf. 2012;21:i9-i12; and The American Board of Pediatrics. Entrustable professional activities for general pediatrics. 2019. Available at: https://www.abp.org/entrustable-professional-activities-epas. Accessed 4 September 2019.

"low value," boring, or irrelevant to the internship/placement experience. Rather, early exposure to telehealth consultations can help normalize such consultations as a core skill in the practice of medicine.

Implementation of the EPA is not discussed in detail here. One avenue we envisage, is the development of a training package suitable as a continuing medical education module to quickly upskill established clinicians who are likely to supervise medical students and residents. In parallel, medical schools could begin to embed telehealth into core curricula (based on the EPA) to prospectively train emerging doctors.

DISCUSSION

Telehealth consultations should be incorporated into core curricula of medical schools, offered during postgraduate years as a core module, and be an entrustable professional activity given the increasing use of telehealth in medical practice and the distinct differences when compared with face-to-face consultations. Competency-based assessments of telephone and video consultations actioned as EPAs not only provide a clear and consistent way for learning and teaching, but also objective appraisal of student and trainee readiness to conduct telehealth consultations with appropriate levels of supervision.

In this article, we focused on competencies for telephone and video consultations by doctors; however, given the increasingly digitized/virtual delivery of health care, these competencies can be used and adapted for other health care professionals offering telehealth consultations, for example, nurse practitioners and clinical pharmacists.

Table 7				
Example of a structured observation tool for formative and/or summative assessment of telephone and video consultations				
Trainee Name and Date:	**NA**	**Poor**	**Competent**	**Excellent**
Preparation				
Conducts consultation in a quiet room with a headset				
Has free hands for taking notes				
Has access to resources that can support clinical decision-making and follow-up actions, for example, electronic health record				
Introduction				
Allows sufficient time for patient/parent[a] to answer the phone/connection				
Checks that the patient/parent is in a private, quiet space, and that it is a convenient time to talk				
Begins by self-introduction and where they are calling from				
Verifies patient's/parent's identity (eg, "To make sure I've reached the right person, could you please say your name, birthday, and address?")				
Avoids putting a call/connection on hold without first assessing the reason for the call				
Information gathering				
Identifies reason for the call (if incoming call)				
Listens attentively to answers and concerns (eg, by using silence skillfully ie, using minimal encouragers eg, "uh-huh" when patient/parent is speaking; and not interrupting)				
Explores patient's/parent's health understanding/beliefs including identifying and addressing patient's ideas, (hidden) concerns and expectations				
Defines the clinical problem				
Explains at the start that several questions may need to be asked to assess their health problem				
Determines the urgency of patient/parent concerns by asking discriminating, open-ended questions and checking for red flags				
Makes an appropriate working diagnosis				
Management plan construction				

(continued on next page)

Table 7 (continued)				
Trainee Name and Date:	**NA**	**Poor**	**Competent**	**Excellent**
Creates an appropriate, effective and mutually acceptable treatment (including medication guidance) and management outcome				
Switches to face-to-face consultation when required (eg, when the diagnosis or management plan cannot be discussed via phone/video consultation, or when an in-person examination may be needed)				
Provides guidance on how to recognize deterioration by describing warning signs and appropriate ensuing actions				
Invites patient/parent to make notes				
Provides suitable education/information resources				
Closure				
Gives a specific window for follow-up (ie, another call) and assesses if these are safe, workable, and appropriate				
Provides explicit safety netting by asking the patient/parent to call back if they have any concerns, if the condition worsens, or does not improve as anticipated				
Recaps key points for the patient/parent				
Checks 2-sided comprehension (by asking the patient/parent to summarize the key points)				
Ends the call by asking if there is anything else the patient/parent is worried about and if the patient/parent has any questions				
Allows the patient/parent to disconnect first				
Effective use of voice and attention				
Uses a clear, warm, non-monotonous tone of voice				
Speaks at a pace that allows clear enunciation of words				
Pays careful attention to (non)verbal and vocal cues, such as silence, (emotional) voice changes, breathing, swallowing and any other sounds				
Confirms that they are still paying attention and on the line by using expressions such as "uh-huh," "OK" when patient/parent is speaking				

(continued on next page)

Table 7 (continued)				
Trainee Name and Date:	**NA**	**Poor**	**Competent**	**Excellent**
Explains sounds in the background when speaking (eg, lets the patient/parent know when making notes to explain the typing sound)				
Additional considerations for video consultations				
Framing and positioning of camera to show trainee's head and shoulders				
Uses neutral background, good lighting				
Makes necessary movement/gestures in view of the camera				
Slows down movement/gestures to avoid blurring on video				
Uses screen share to show images/ diagnostic findings to patient				
Management of group interactions of those present at the video consultation that is, patient, parents, family				
Awareness of and preparedness to activate virtual care pathways (eg, emergency and urgent care centers in the patient's local area)				

[a] In the case of young children, the parent/caregiver/family are mediators of the telehealth consultation. However, the trainee should engage directly with the child when appropriate to do so.

We described the development and pilot of a telehealth training program, and proposed an EPA for telehealth for further refinement and discussion, as a contribution to the field. In medicine, an ACGME curriculum for telemedicine has been proposed for neurology residents,[38] whereas other health professions, such as nursing and pharmacy, are also beginning to publish guidelines and offer similar training.[39–41]

Future Research

Amidst the various telehealth training across different health professions (not to mention those offered commercially), there is a need for an overarching quality and safety framework to ascertain the robustness of training programs, and whether training translates to effective skills. In addition, Hilty and colleagues[42] argue for a need to evaluate telehealth competency frameworks across various health care professions, to ensure a consistent quality of care using this modality. Telehealth itself is evolving in its modes of delivery, scope, and nature. Hence, training should keep pace with these technological trends and innovations, such as the increasing use of AI in conjunction.

Limitations

We have assumed the availability of suitably trained supervisors to assess trainees' competency in telehealth consultations; that patient selection is appropriate and prudent; that Internet connectivity and reasonable broadband speeds are available (for video consultations), but acknowledge that in some locations this is not the case due to infrastructure limitations. We have also assumed that patients are able to easily access and can afford equipment necessary for telehealth consultations. In framing telehealth training as extended communication skills, existing criticisms regarding the teaching and assessment of clinical communication skills apply.[43]

SUMMARY

The future of health care delivery is inseparable from telehealth. Emerging and practicing doctors need to acquire telehealth consultation skills to thrive in the increasingly pressurized health system of delivering high-quality, high-volume health care with a shrinking health care workforce. The use of competency-based training for telehealth, operationalized as an entrustable professional activity, could ensure high-quality, safe, and effective telehealth consultations.

AUTHOR CONTRIBUTIONS

E. Lum conceptualized the article; drafted, and critically revised the article; reviewed the learning objectives and training manual for the pilot telehealth training workshop; mapped the learning objectives to the ACGME and CanMEDS competency frameworks; and developed the proposed EPA for telehealth. L.S. van Galen conceptualized and developed the telehealth training learning objectives and training manuals (including case scenarios, presentations, formative assessment tool, and feedback surveys); delivered the pilot telehealth training workshop; and provided critical review of the article. J. Car conceived the idea for the article; supervised E. Lum and L.S. van Galen; and critically revised the article.

DISCLOSURE

The authors have nothing to disclose.

REFERENCES

1. Guttman D. 29 statistics you need to know about healthcare & telemedicine. 2017. Available at: https://www.fshealth.com/blog/29-statistics-about-telemedicine-healthcare. Accessed September 4, 2019.
2. van Galen L, Car J. Telephone consultations. BMJ 2018;360:k1047. Available at: https://www.ncbi.nlm.nih.gov/pubmed/29599197.
3. Reismann AB, Stevens DL. Telephone medicine: a guide for the practicing physician. Philadelphia: American College of Physicians; 2002.
4. Schmitt BD. Pediatric telephone protocols: office version. 15th edition. Itasca, IL: American Academy of Pediatrics; 2016.
5. Thompson DA. Adult telephone protocols: office version. 3rd edition. Itasca, IL: American Academy of Pediatrics; 2013.
6. Car J, Sheikh A. Telephone consultations. BMJ 2003;326(7396):966–9. Available at: https://www.bmj.com/content/326/7396/966.
7. Kim J, Bea W, Lee K, et al. Effect of the telephone-delivered nutrition education on dietary intake and biochemical parameters in subjects with metabolic syndrome. Clin Nutr Res 2013;2(2):115–24. Available at: https://www.ncbi.nlm.nih.gov/pubmed/23908978.
8. Banbury A, Nancarrow S, Dart J, et al. Telehealth interventions delivering home-based support group videoconferencing: systematic review. J Med Internet Res 2018;20(2): e25. Available at: https://www.ncbi.nlm.nih.gov/pmc/articles/PMC5816261/.
9. Smith AC, Scuffham P, Wootton R. The costs and potential savings of a novel tele-paediatric service in Queensland. BMC Health Serv Res 2007;7(35). https://doi.org/

10.1186/1472-6963-7-35. Available at: https://bmchealthservres.biomedcentral.com/articles/10.1186/1472-6963-7-35.

10. Brownlee GL, Caffery LJ, McBride CA, et al. Telehealth in paediatric surgery: accuracy of clinical decisions made by videoconference. J Paediatr Child Health 2017;53(12):1220–5. Available at: https://www.ncbi.nlm.nih.gov/pubmed/28589677.

11. Utidjian L, Abramson E. Pediatric telehealth: opportunities and challenges. Pediatr Clin North Am 2016;63(2):367–78. Available at: https://www.ncbi.nlm.nih.gov/pubmed/27017042.

12. Bradford NK, Caffery LJ, Taylor M, et al. Speech-language pathology services delivered by telehealth in a rural educational setting: the school's perspective. J Int Soc Telemed eHealth 2018;6. https://doi.org/10.29086/JISfTeH.6.e20. Available at: https://journals.ukzn.ac.za/index.php/JISfTeH/article/view/719.

13. Dorsey ER, Topol EJ. State of telehealth. N Engl J Med 2016;375(2):154–61. https://doi.org/10.1056/NEJMra1601705. Available at:.

14. Dullet NW, Geraghty EM, Kaufman T, et al. Impact of a university-based outpatient telemedicine program on time savings, travel costs, and environmental pollutants. Value Health 2017;20(4):542–6. Available at: https://www.ncbi.nlm.nih.gov/pubmed/28407995.

15. Ranjan P, Kumari A, Chakrawarty A. How can doctors improve their communication skills? J Clin Diagn Res 2015;9(3):JE01–4. Available at: https://www.ncbi.nlm.nih.gov/pmc/articles/PMC4413084/.

16. Rimmer A. How do I improve my communication skills? BMJ 2017;357:j2587. Available at: https://www.bmj.com/content/357/bmj.j2587.

17. Boudreau JD, Cassell E, Fuks A. Preparing medical students to become attentive listeners. Med Teach 2009;31(1):22–9.

18. Lussier M-T, Richard C. Doctor-patient communication: complaints and legal actions. Can Fam Physician 2005;51(1):37–9. Available at: https://www.ncbi.nlm.nih.gov/pmc/articles/PMC1479583/.

19. van Galen L, Wang C, Nanayakkara P, et al. Telehealth requires expansion of physicians' communication competencies training. Med Teach 2019;41(6):714–5. Available at: https://www.ncbi.nlm.nih.gov/pubmed/29944031.

20. American Medical Association. Telehealth up 53%, growing faster than any other place of care. 2019. Available at: https://www.ama-assn.org/practice-management/digital/telehealth-53-growing-faster-any-other-place-care. Accessed September 4, 2019.

21. Sharma R, Nachum S, Davidson KW, et al. It's not just FaceTime: core competencies for the medical virtualist. Int J Emerg Med 2019;12(8). https://doi.org/10.1186/s12245-019-0226-y.

22. Olson CA, McSwain SD, Curfman AL, et al. The current pediatric telehealth landscape. Pediatrics 2018;141(3):e20172334.

23. Elnicki DM, Ogden P, Flannery M, et al. Telephone medicine for internists. J Gen Intern Med 2000;15(5):337–43. Available at: https://www.ncbi.nlm.nih.gov/pmc/articles/PMC1495459/.

24. Katz HP, Kaltsounis D, Halloran L, et al. Patient safety and telephone medicine: some lessons from closed claim case review. J Gen Intern Med 2008;23(5):517–22. Available at: https://www.ncbi.nlm.nih.gov/pmc/articles/PMC2324141/.

25. Hannis MD, Elnicki DM, Morris DK, et al. Can you hold please? How internal medicine residents deal with patient telephone calls. Telephone Encounters Learning Initiative Group. Am J Med Sci 1994;308(6):349–52. Available at: https://www.ncbi.nlm.nih.gov/pubmed/7985723.

26. Derkx HP, Rethans JJ, Maiburg BH, et al. Quality of communication during telephone triage at Dutch out-of-hours centres. Patient Educ Couns 2009;74(2): 174–8. Available at: https://www.ncbi.nlm.nih.gov/pubmed/18845413.

27. Car J, Freeman GK, Partridge MR, et al. Improving quality and safety of telephone based delivery of care: teaching telephone consultation skills. BMJ Qual Saf 2004;13(1):2–3. Available at: https://www.ncbi.nlm.nih.gov/pmc/articles/PMC1758049/pdf/v013p00002.pdf.

28. Bunn F, Byrne G, Kendall S. Telephone consultation and triage: effects on health care use and patient satisfaction. Cochrane Database Syst Rev 2004;(4). CD004180. Available at: http://onlinelibrary.wiley.com/doi/10.1002/14651858. CD004180.pub2/abstract.

29. Vaona A, Pappas Y, Grewal RS, et al. Training interventions for improving telephone consultation skills in clinicians. Cochrane Database Syst Rev 2017;(1). CD010034. Available at: http://onlinelibrary.wiley.com/doi/10.1002/14651858. CD010034.pub2/abstract.

30. Medical Protection Practice Matters. Risk of telephone consultations. 2015. Available at: https://www.medicalprotection.org/uk/practice-matters-june-2015/risks-of-telephone-consultations. Accessed September 13, 2019.

31. Holmboe ES, Edgar L, Hamstra S. The milestones guidebook. Chicago, IL: Accreditation Council for Graduate Medical Education; 2016.

32. Royal College of Physicians and Surgeons of Canada. CanMEDS: better standards, better physicians, better care. 2019. Available at: http://www.royalcollege.ca/rcsite/canmeds/canmeds-framework-e. Accessed September 6, 2019.

33. ten Cate O, Young JQ. The patient handover as an entrustable professional activity: adding meaning in teaching and practice. BMJ Qual Saf 2012;21:i9–12. Available at: https://qualitysafety.bmj.com/content/21/Suppl_1/i9.

34. Lum E, Mitchell C, Coombes I. The competent prescriber: 12 core competencies for safe prescribing. Aust Prescr 2013;36(1):13–6. Available at: https://www.nps.org.au/australian-prescriber/articles/the-competent-prescriber-12-core-competencies-for-safe-prescribing.

35. The American Board of Pediatrics. Entrustable professional activities for general pediatrics. 2019. Available at: https://www.abp.org/entrustable-professional-activities-epas. Accessed September 4, 2019.

36. The American Board of Pediatrics. Entrustable professional activities for subspecialties. 2019. Available at: https://www.abp.org/subspecialty-epas. Accessed September 4, 2019.

37. El-Haddad C, Damodaran A, McNeil H, et al. The ABCs of entrustable professional activities: an overview of 'entrustable professional activities' in medical education. Intern Med J 2016;46(9):1006–10. Available at: https://www.ncbi.nlm.nih.gov/pubmed/26388198.

38. Baruchin A. A proposed ACGME curriculum in telemedicine for neurology residents. 2017. Available at: https://journals.lww.com/neurotodayonline/FullText/2017/08170/Professionalism__A_Proposed_ACGME_Curriculum_in.1.aspx. Accessed September 3, 2019.

39. Badowski ME, Walker S, Bacchus S, et al. Providing comprehensive medication management in telehealth. Pharmacotherapy 2018;38(2):e7–16. Available at: https://www.ncbi.nlm.nih.gov/pubmed/29239004.

40. Rutledge CM, Kott K, Schweickert PA, et al. Telehealth and eHealth in nurse practitioner training: current perspectives. Adv Med Educ Pract 2017;8:399–409. Available at: https://www.ncbi.nlm.nih.gov/pmc/articles/PMC5498674/.

41. van Houwelingen CT, Moerman AH, Ettema RG, et al. Competencies required for nursing telehealth activities: a Delphi study. Nurse Educ Today 2016;39:50–62. Available at: https://www.sciencedirect.com/science/article/pii/ S0260691716000149?via%3Dihub.

42. Hilty DM, Maheu MM, Drude KP, et al. The need to implement and evaluate telehealth competency frameworks to ensure quality care across behavioral health professions. Acad Psychiatry 2018;42:818–24.

43. Salmon P, Young B. Creativity in clinical communication: from communication skills to skilled communication. Med Educ 2011;45:217–26. Available at: https://www.ncbi.nlm.nih.gov/pubmed/21299597.

44. World Health Organization. Health and sustainable development. 2019. Available at: https://www.who.int/sustainable-development/health-sector/strategies/telehealth/ en/. Accessed September 3, 2019.

45. ten Cate O. Nuts and bolts of entrustable professional activities. J Grad Med Educ 2013;157–8. https://doi.org/10.4300/JGME-D-12-00380.1.

46. ten Cate O. A primer on entrustable professional activities. Korean J Med Educ 2018;30(1):1–10.

47. Mink RB, Schwartz A, Herman BE, et al. Validity of level of supervision scales for assessing pediatric fellows on the common pediatric subspecialty entrustable professional activities. Acad Med 2018;93(2):283–91. Available at: https://www. ncbi.nlm.nih.gov/pubmed/28700462.

Tele-rounds and Case-Based Training

Project ECHO Telementoring Model Applied to Complex Diabetes Care

Nicolas Cuttriss, MD, MPH[a],*, Matthew F. Bouchonville, MD[b],
David M. Maahs, MD, PhD[c], Ashby F. Walker, PhD[d]

KEYWORDS

- Telehealth • Distance education • Diabetes • Type 1 diabetes • Insulin
- Vulnerable populations • Care delivery • Project ECHO

KEY POINTS

- Project ECHO (Extension for Community Healthcare Outcomes) is a low-dose, high-frequency workforce development model of education and guided practice that leverages videoconferencing technology to connect specialists with learners across geographic distances.
- Diabetes is a complex chronic medical condition and insulin management further adds to the complexity of medical management in the primary care setting.
- Workforce shortages of endocrinologists and barriers to receiving specialty care for patients with diabetes mandates innovative health care delivery solutions to amplify and democratize specialty knowledge.
- T1D incidence is increasing with the largest burden of disease in the adult population; efforts to address improvement in health care delivery are required across the lifespan.
- The ECHO model is a telementoring model that can be applied to T1D to address disparities and urgent needs of complex patients throughout the lifespan.

[a] Division of Endocrinology, Department of Pediatrics, Stanford University School of Medicine, Stanford, CA, USA; [b] Division of Endocrinology, Diabetes and Metabolism, University of New Mexico, MSC10 5550 1 University of New Mexico, Albuquerque, NM 87131, USA; [c] Division of Endocrinology, Department of Pediatrics, Stanford University School of Medicine, 300 Pasteur Drive, Room G-313, Stanford, CA 94305, USA; [d] Department of Health Services Research, Management and Policy, HPNP, Room 3117, University of Florida, Gainesville, FL 32611, USA
* Corresponding author. Department of Pediatrics, Division of Endocrinology and Diabetes, Stanford University School of Medicine, 300 Pasteur Drive, Room G-313 Medical Center, Stanford, CA 94305, USA.
E-mail address: cuttriss@stanford.edu

Pediatr Clin N Am 67 (2020) 759–772
https://doi.org/10.1016/j.pcl.2020.04.017
0031-3955/20/© 2020 Elsevier Inc. All rights reserved.

pediatric.theclinics.com

INTRODUCTION

Medical knowledge is often limited among too few specialists and the flow of specialty medical knowledge to patients is further limited by the lack of supply of specialists (**Fig. 1**). With respect to diabetes, there is a workforce shortage of endocrinologists and diabetes specialists in the United States[1–4] and in low- and middle-income countries that is resulting in primary care providers (PCPs) needing to take on the role of the diabetes specialists.[5,6] This supply shortage is further compounded by the increasing incidence in diabetes[7,8] and decline in providers pursuing diabetes specialization within endocrinology.[9]

Diabetes is a complex chronic medical condition and insulin management further adds to the complexity of medical management in the primary care setting. The prevalence and incidence of diabetes, type 1 diabetes (T1D) and type 2 diabetes (T2D), is increasing at alarming rates in the United States and globally.[7,10,11] More than 450 million people globally have diabetes and one-quarter to one-half of that population are estimated to require insulin.[12–14] Insulin is required for all forms of T1D, which accounts for an estimated 30 million people worldwide and 5% of the 30.3 million people in the United States living with diabetes.[10,11,15]

Focus of T1D management in the primary care setting provides the opportunity to assess needs and barriers to intensive insulin therapy among PCPs managing patients with complex diabetes requiring insulin. T1D is the most common chronic endocrinological condition in childhood. Although T1D is often seen as a pediatric condition with the most newly diagnosed cases occurring in the pediatric age group, the largest burden and prevalence of T1D is in the adult population.[7,8,11,16] Innovative efforts to address improvements in health care delivery for T1D are required across the lifespan and not just in pediatrics.

More frequent diabetes team visits and touch points for patients with T1D have been demonstrated to improve glycemic targets and reduce risk of microvascular and

Work & Income:
For low-income children with T1D, financial barriers for parents like time lost from work may be an obstacle.

Access and Workforce Shortage:
For adults with T1D, there is a critical and growing shortage of adult endocrinologists.

Distance & Rural Obstacles:
'For children and adults with T1D in rural areas, distance may be an obstacle.

Beyond distance:
For adults and children with T1D who are in close proximity to endocrinologists, barriers other than distance persist.

Fig. 1. Barriers to receiving specialty endocrinology care in type 1 diabetes (T1D). (Reprinted with permission from *Project ECHO T1D Research Group*.)

cardiovascular complications.[17,18] The American Diabetes Association–recommended routine follow-up care is quarterly visits in patients with T1D and quarterly to semiannually visits in patients with T2D.[19,20] However, this is not possible within current health care delivery systems because there are not enough endocrinologists to see all patients with diabetes annually, let alone quarterly.[1] Geographic and socioeconomic considerations further limit the practicality of patients with T1D to receive quarterly in-person follow-up visits. It is particularly crucial to implement programs that address the barriers high-need, high-cost patients with T1D face in receiving routine diabetes care.[21]

Telemedicine initiatives within diabetes specialty centers are promising in their ability to improve access, continuity of care, patient satisfaction, and outcomes.[22–24] However, an undefined percentage of the pediatric and adult population are unable to use diabetes specialty centers and rely on nonspecialty care for routine or urgent care related to their diabetes. To address disparities and barriers to receiving specialty care in T1D, specialty knowledge in diabetes needs to be democratized from specialists to frontline PCPs. Project ECHO (Extension for Community Healthcare Outcomes) telementoring model is an example of an approach to do so within diabetes, and more specifically the subset of diabetes population with T1D requiring complex care and insulin management.

EXTENSION FOR COMMUNITY HEALTHCARE OUTCOMES MODEL

The ECHO model is a "hub-and-spoke" outreach telementoring model committed to addressing the needs of the most vulnerable populations who do not have access to specialists by creating learning loops by moving knowledge to community practitioners instead of moving patients to specialty centers. Through the use of technology, education, and research, Project ECHO democratizes specialty knowledge and amplifies the capacity for PCPs to provide best practice care to their patients.[25,26] The model uses case-based learning, essentially applying the same learning methodologies used by medical student and residency training programs. The usual format of a teleECHO session involves weekly to monthly conferencing meetings where community health care professionals "present" deidentified patients to the ECHO learning network, consisting of ECHO specialists and community peers, and receive ongoing guidance in management. Over the course of regular participation, community health care professionals develop the expertise and confidence to manage higher complexity patients with less need for referrals to a specialist. Additionally, best practices are disseminated across the learning network in a multidirectional fashion as new evidence emerges (**Fig. 2**).

The model was developed out of the University of New Mexico Health Sciences Center in 2003, for hepatitis C by Dr Sanjeev Arora in response to the (1) lack of access to hepatitis C virus (HCV) specialists and long wait times, (2) high treatment failure rates, and (3) lack of confidence among community practitioners in managing or comanaging HCV. The model demonstrated improved patient outcomes in HCV cure rates, particularly among the medically vulnerable.[26,27]

Project ECHO has since been expanded from HCV to more than 70 specialty medical conditions, including endocrinology and diabetes, and replicated and adapted at more than 360 hub sites globally.[28] Replication of the model has been achieved by identifying and training ECHO "hubs" (regional specialty centers) who partner with "spokes" (regional clinic sites). Hence, new capacity for complex disease management has been rapidly developed around the globe where access to specialty care is limited. As with complex diabetes care,[29,30] medical conditions that are

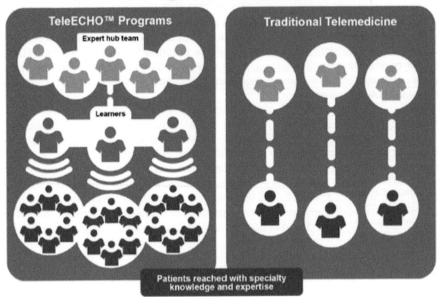

Fig. 2. Project ECHO is not traditional telemedicine and leverages telementoring to interact with groups of providers to amplify knowledge and the effect of the specialist. (Reprinted with permission from Project ECHO®/ECHO Institute™.)

appropriately managed through the ECHO model exhibit the following six characteristics: (1) the disease is common, (2) management of the disease is complex, (3) treatment of the disease is evolving, (4) the disease has high societal impact, (5) there are serious consequences of not treating the disease, and (6) improved outcomes are obtained with disease management.[25] Accordingly, the ECHO model of workforce development through guided practice may be generalizable to numerous chronic diseases.

The ECHO model differs from traditional telemedicine and telehealth in particular in that it has an amplification effect and addresses the underlying lack of specialists to demonopolize specialty knowledge (**Table 1**). As illustrated in **Fig. 3**, the model builds capacity and specialty knowledge among community providers by: (1) using technology to leverage scarce resources and create knowledge networks by connecting spokes (learners from community provider sites) with hub (multidisciplinary team of experts at regional center) through regularly scheduled teleECHO sessions using Zoom or alternative communications platform; (2) improving outcomes by sharing best practices and reducing variations in processes of care; (3) case-based learning that facilitates learning loops, democratizes specialty knowledge, and self-efficacy among nonspecialists; and (4) program evaluation and data tracking for quality improvement.[25,28]

Application of Extension for Community Healthcare Outcomes Model to Type 1 Diabetes

Applying the ECHO model, Stanford University and the University of Florida Diabetes Institute (UFDI) partnered with the ECHO Institute at the University of New Mexico Health Sciences Center to develop and pilot the model for T1D (Project ECHO T1D)

Table 1
Distinguishing features of TeleECHO, Telehealth, and Telemedicine

Feature	TeleECHO	Telehealth	Telemedicine
Hub and spoke model	✔	✔	
Videoconferencing/Internet	✔	✔	✔
Underserved populations	✔	✔	✔
Case consultation	✔	✔	✔
Doctor-patient relationship			✔
Coverage of services (CPT codes)			✔
Remote patient monitoring			✔
Patients are deidentified	✔	✔	
Case-based learning	✔	✔	
Brief lectures	✔	✔	
Continuing education/continuing medical education credits	✔	✔	
Learning loops to develop subspecialty expertise overtime	✔		
"Demonopolizes" specialty knowledge	✔		

Adapted from ECHO Institute Replication Guide and with permission from Project ECHO/ECHO Institute.

Four Principles of the ECHO Model

Use Technology to leverage scarce resources

Share "best practices" to reduce disparities

Apply case-based learning to master complexity

Evaluate and monitor outcomes

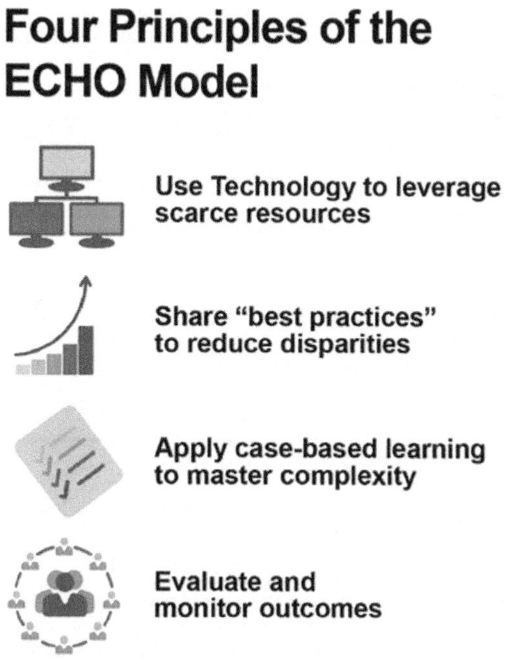

Fig. 3. Principles of Project ECHO model. (Reprinted with permission from Project ECHO®/ECHO Institute™.)

in the states of California and Florida. The goal of the pilot was to demonstrate the feasibility of an ECHO model for T1D and improve the ability of PCPs to manage patients with T1D (**Fig. 4**).

Identifying barriers and needs

Before launching and piloting Project ECHO T1D teleECHO program, Stanford and the UFDI teams conducted needs assessment to identify barriers and needs of PCP and patients with T1D who do not routinely see endocrinologists (**Fig. 5**).

Survey research was conducted with PCP community providers in California and Florida using publicly available provider directories (n = 123; response rate 55% in California and 44% in Florida). PCP surveys asked about basic protocols for T1D care, insulin prescribing habits, referral patterns, confidence in insulin and diabetes management, and potential interest in Project ECHO T1D. Findings highlighted lack of PCP confidence in insulin management despite high prescribing habits of insulin in pediatric and adult populations.[31]

Focus groups (n = 18) were conducted in California and Florida among vulnerable patients with T1D 18 years and older to identify barriers to care among adults with T1D who do not receive routine specialty endocrinology care. Barriers to care reported included: (1) cost of insulin and supplies, (2) long wait times when needing to schedule adult endocrinology visits, (3) lack of attention to T1D care during adult endocrinology visits, (4) distance required to travel to specialist, (5) preference to defer to their PCP over endocrinologist for T1D care, and (6) lack of local support groups for T1D or networks therein.[6,31]

Findings from the PCP survey research and patient focus groups were used to further develop Project ECHO T1D curriculum and develop the TeleECHO program (**Fig. 6**).

Developing project Extension for Community Healthcare Outcomes program and spoke recruitment

Hub team formation A multidisciplinary team approach to supporting diverse needs of complex patients with chronic disease and T1D has been demonstrated to improve health outcomes.[32,33] Multidisciplinary hub team members (adult endocrinologist, pediatric endocrinologists, behavior health specialist, diabetes educator, pharmacist,

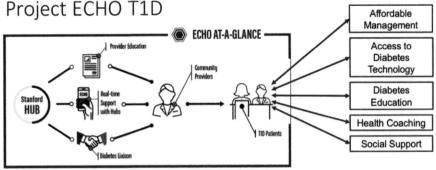

Goal: Increase the capacity of primary care providers and clinics to empower and safely and effectively manage underserved patients with T1D who do not receive routine specialty care.

Opportunity: Leverage other resources into Project ECHO T1D to patients with T1D.

Fig. 4. Overview of Project ECHO T1D model.

Project ECHO T1D Phases

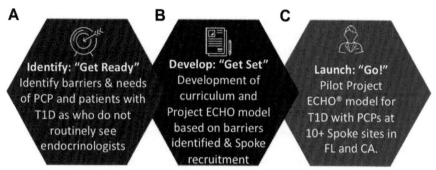

A

Identify: "Get Ready"
Identify barriers & needs of PCP and patients with T1D as who do not routinely see endocrinologists

B

Develop: "Get Set"
Development of curriculum and Project ECHO model based on barriers identified & Spoke recruitment

C

Launch: "Go!"
Pilot Project ECHO® model for T1D with PCPs at 10+ Spoke sites in FL and CA.

Fig. 5. Phases of the initial 18-month pilot program of Project ECHO T1D.

- Survey research conducted with PCP community providers in CA and FL
- Results highlighted lack of PCP confidence in insulin management despite high prescribing habits of insulin in pediatric and adult populations

Primary Care Provider Needs Assessment: Survey Research

- Focus groups conducted with patients with T1D in CA and FL
- Barriers to care identified amongst adults with T1D who do not receive routine specialty endocrinology care

T1D Patient Needs Assessment: Focus Groups

- Geocoding of PCPs and endocrinologists using the Neighborhood Deprivation Index (NDI) to identify high-need geographic catchment areas for T1D patients
- Insurance claims data used to identify PCPs treating T1D
- Survey data from PCPs needs assessment
- Word-of-moth interest
- Site visits to interested spoke sites
- Pilot spoke sites selected and "T1D Champion" identified at each spoke site
- Collaboration agreements signed between hub-and-spoke sites

Precision Spoke Recruitment

- Identification of specialists to serve on multidisciplinary hub teams
- Training and travel of hub teams to ECHO Institute for "ECHO Immersion" training
- Evaluation and program plan developed
- Curriculum developed by hub teams with feedback from spoke sites
- Continuing education (CE, CME) application and approval
- In-person orientation and training of T1D champions from spoke sites

TeleECHO & Curriculum Development

Fig. 6. Summary of methodology used in developing Project ECHO T1D teleECHO program. CA, California; FL, Florida.

T1D health coaches) were identified and recruited at each hub site to join the Project ECHO T1D team. Hub team members participated in the ECHO Institute's 3-day "Immersion Training" program in Albuquerque, New Mexico. Hub team members agreed to mentor spoke sites and provide care management recommendations during teleECHO sessions. Hub team members were allotted 5% to 10% protected time to participate in Project ECHO T1D. In addition, a clinic coordinator (100% **full-time equivalent (FTE)**)) and clinic director (50% FTE) were allocated dedicated protected time to support the development and launch the program. The UFDI and Stanford hub teams held weekly steering committee videoconference calls to share best practices and coordinate implementation.

Spoke site recruitment Spoke sites were recruited targeting vulnerable T1D patient populations more likely to rely on PCPs for diabetes care as a result of lack of access or use of routine specialty endocrinology care. Precision spoke recruitment methods included: (1) geocoding using the Neighborhood Deprivation Index to identify high-need areas, (2) claims data from select payers to identify PCPs treating T1D, and (3) analysis of results collected from PCP needs assessments surveys. federally qualified health centers were also targeted. The clinic coordinator and clinic director from each hub site traveled and met face-to-face with interested spoke sites and identified an "ECHO T1D clinic champion" at each spoke site to serve as lead staff representative for the clinic. Other health care providers or other nonclinician staff team members were also encouraged to work with the champion and participate in the weekly teleECHO sessions. Collaboration agreements between the hub team and each respective spoke sites were signed before commencement of the teleECHO program. In California, 11 spoke sites enrolled with 37 clinics serving roughly 900 adult and pediatric patients with T1D who do not receive specialty T1D care. In Florida, 12 spoke sites enrolled with 67 clinics who serve roughly 1300 patients with T1D (**Fig. 7**).

Curriculum development A 6-month curriculum of weekly brief (15–20 minutes) lecture sessions and a subsequent 6-month curriculum of alternating weekly lectures was developed by the hub teams with feedback from spoke sites. Educational needs

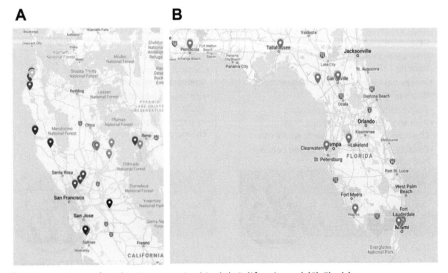

Fig. 7. Locations of spoke sites recruited in (A) California and (B) Florida.

assessment and preferred topics were surveyed among spoke sites before the start and throughout the program. Spoke feedback was incorporated into the curriculum and flexibility was integrated into the curriculum to allow for "topics on demand." Continuing education (CE) and continuing medical education (CME) applications were submitted and approved at both hub sites. Hub teams had option of offering CE/CME through the University of New Mexico or through respective institutions. Lecture sessions were recorded and archived for spokes. Some examples of sessions include: T1D Versus T2D, Making a Diagnosis of T1D in Primary Care, Initiating Insulin and Dose Calculation, Types of Insulin Analogues, Blood Glucose Monitoring, Continuous Glucose Monitoring Systems, Carbohydrate Counting and Dietary Management in T1D, Screening for Depression and Diabetes Burnout, Diabulimia and Disordered Eating, Motivational Interviewing, Introducing Diabetes Technology to Patients, Insulin Pumps, Screening for Comorbidities and Complications, Adjunct T1D Therapy, Pre-Conception Counseling and T1D Management During Pregnancy, PCOS and T1D, Transitioning From Pediatric to Adult Care, Knowing Patient Rights: Diabetes in the Workplace, Affording T1D Prescriptions, and Diabetes Disparities.

Diabetes liaison and type 1 diabetes health coach The traditional ECHO model encourages spoke sites to incorporate community health workers into the program model and to be active participants at the spoke sites.[34] The Project ECHO T1D model recruits persons living with T1D or family members of persons living with T1D in the community to serve as diabetes liaisons (ie, T1D health coaches) to provide additional social support services to patients with T1D at spoke sites. This additional resource is offered as an opt-in service to spoke sites and personnel are hired and trained by the hub team. Patients with T1D who are interested in the nonmedical advice services (telephone calls, home visits, care navigation, social gatherings with others with T1D) are able to opt-in to the T1D health coach program via a social contract.

Launching Project ECHO T1D TeleECHO program
Benefits to the spoke sites in participating in the teleECHO program include:

- *In-person training and orientation:* 2-day training program to orient and build community of practice among spokes and hub.
- *TeleECHO sessions:* dedicated hour-long, weekly telementoring clinic for community practices to present challenging T1D cases for recommendations to multidisciplinary team.
- *Real-time support:* hub team provides spokes with access to real-time support during off-hours of teleECHO sessions.
- *Diabetes liaison (ie, T1D health coach):* additional social support services available to spokes that enables patients with T1D to opt-in via a social contract.
- *Clinical research access:* opportunities to enroll patients in clinical research opportunities and initiatives at the hub.
- *Continuing education:* spoke participants receive no cost American Medical Association CME and CE credits.
- *Sponsorship:* spoke participation in program free of charge and spokes also receive small stipend for pilot phase participation.

The Stanford and UFDI hub teams facilitated dedicated weekly hour-long telementoring sessions for spokes sites throughout the states of California and Florida. A teleECHO session is demonstrated in **Fig. 8**. Spoke site participation was organized and led by the ECHO T1D clinic champion but was open to any provider or team member at the spoke site. As demonstrated in **Table 2**, each hour-long teleECHO session

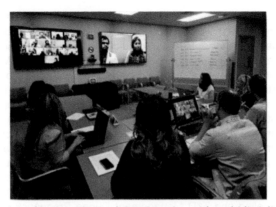

Fig. 8. Demonstration of Project ECHO teleECHO session with multidisciplinary hub team in-person and representatives from spoke sites remotely joining clinic via Zoom platform. (Reprinted with permission from Project ECHO®/ECHO Institute™.)

includes (1) introduction and announcements, (2) brief lecture, (3) case presentations, and (4) questions and answers. The program schedule changes to alternating weekly sessions after 6 months of weekly teleECHOs.

Table 2
Sample teleECHO session agenda

Time Allocation	Session Agenda Item	Comments
10 min	Introductions and announcements	Weekly attendance recorded in chat box and by video introductions and later uploaded into iECHO evaluation system for monitoring and evaluation
15–20 min	Brief lectures	Curriculum developed in collaboration with learners to address topics of highest interest and least confidence
15–30 min	Case presentation 1	Deidentified case presentation form submitted online (RedCap survey) by spoke site at least 2 d before session. Spoke site representative presents case to network of hub and spokes and solicits feedback. New case presentations that are complex may take up to 30 min and this allows for discretion of clinic director to limit to 1 case presentation per week
10–15 min	Case presentation 2	Represent cases are encouraged and less time allocated for the represents
5 min	Questions and answers	Multidisciplinary recommendations are summarized at end of each teleECHO session and then posted online for reference. Evaluation and continuing education links e-mailed to attendees after session

A teleECHO program is an all-teach all-learn mentoring program that builds community of practice over time. Before each teleECHO session, spoke sites upload deidentified case presentations for discussion. Recommendations are provided by other spoke sites in addition to the multidisciplinary hub team. Project ECHO T1D staff review case presentations, administer surveys, coordinate CME, support spoke site needs, support patient needs through T1D health coaches, and work to make Project ECHO T1D sustainable. Project ECHO T1D staff are available Monday through Friday to field administrative and clinical inquiries. During off-hours of the teleECHO program, hub team members are accessible to provide spokes with access to real-time support. Additional off-hour support includes access to participant-only Web site with recordings of brief lectures and toolkits, e-mail support, and telephone support.

DISCUSSION

Persistently suboptimal outcomes for people with diabetes and a lack of access to subspecialty care mandates the development of innovative health care delivery models.[35] With the growing supply-demand mismatch of diabetes specialists compounded by underlying social determinants of health barriers to accessing and using diabetes specialty care, the health care delivery system is in need of interventions that multiply provider efficacy. A telementoring model, such as Project ECHO, can amplify specialty knowledge and minimize barriers to specialty care by building and leveraging local capacity.[27,30,36]

Project ECHO T1D demonstrated feasibility of the ECHO model applied to T1D and improved the ability of PCPs to manage patients with T1D. Enrollment in Project ECHO T1D demonstrated feasibility with extremely high interest among PCPs because the pilot program filled beyond capacity reaching clinics in remote and medically underserved regions.

Focus on T1D served to assess implementation of the ECHO model for diabetes and target PCPs managing insulin. Given most insulin-requiring patients have T2D and therapeutic inertia in T2D is posing a public health dilemma, expansion of the ECHO T1D model to include insulin-requiring patients with T2D is a necessary population health approach.[37–39]

The initiative is now being expanded in scale to support additional clinics throughout California and Florida, and in scope beyond T1D to support PCPs managing all forms of diabetes requiring insulin use (ie, ECHO Diabetes). Stanford and the University of Florida are now preparing to evaluate patient-level outcomes and value considerations for payers, clinics, and providers before preparing for broader implementation of ECHO Diabetes.[40]

Additional academic and nonacademic centers are developing Project ECHO tele-ECHO programs related to endocrinology and diabetes nationally and internationally. Implementation of the Project ECHO T1D model is also currently underway in Ecuador. To date, there are 21 programs across 24 centers in four countries with endocrinology-related Project ECHO programs, which vary in scope.[28] Stanford, UFDI, and the ECHO Institute are also committed to further exploring ways to strengthen the network of diabetes-related Project ECHO programs and scale the model to amplify and democratize specialty knowledge.

ACKNOWLEDGMENTS

The Leona M. and Harry B. Helmsley Charitable Trust generously supported this research.

DISCLOSURE

The authors have nothing to disclose.

REFERENCES

1. Lu H, Holt JB, Cheng YJ, et al. Population-based geographic access to endocrinologists in the United States, 2012. BMC Health Serv Res 2015;15:541.
2. Rizza RA, Vigersky RA, Rodbard HW, et al. A model to determine workforce needs for endocrinologists in the United States until 2020. Diabetes Care 2003; 26(5):1545–52.
3. Stewart AF. The United States endocrinology workforce: a supply-demand mismatch. J Clin Endocrinol Metab 2008;93(4):1164–6.
4. Vigersky RA, Fish L, Hogan P, et al. The clinical endocrinology workforce: current status and future projections of supply and demand. J Clin Endocrinol Metab 2014;99(9):3112–21.
5. Shi L. The impact of primary care: a focused review. Scientifica (Cairo) 2012; 2012:432892.
6. Walker AF, Cuttriss N, Haller MJ, et al. 1265-P: the paradox of care delivery for type 1 diabetes in primary care settings: a call for interventions to reduce health disparities. Diabetes 2019;68(Supplement 1):1265.
7. Krug EG. Trends in diabetes: sounding the alarm. Lancet 2016;387(10027): 1485–6.
8. Maahs DM, West NA, Lawrence JM, et al. Epidemiology of type 1 diabetes. Endocrinol Metab Clin North Am 2010;39(3):481–97.
9. (AAMC) AoAMC. The 2019 update: the complexities of physician supply and demand: projections from 2017 to 2032. Washington , DC: Association of American Medical Colleges; 2019.
10. Imperatore G, Boyle JP, Thompson TJ, et al. Projections of type 1 and type 2 diabetes burden in the U.S. population aged <20 years through 2050: dynamic modeling of incidence, mortality, and population growth. Diabetes Care 2012; 35(12):2515–20.
11. Mayer-Davis EJ, Lawrence JM, Dabelea D, et al. Incidence trends of type 1 and type 2 diabetes among youths, 2002-2012. N Engl J Med 2017;376(15):1419–29.
12. Garg SK, Rewers AH, Akturk HK. Ever-increasing insulin-requiring patients globally. Diabetes Technol Ther 2018;20(S2). S2-S1–S2-4.
13. Basu S, Yudkin JS, Kehlenbrink S, et al. Estimation of global insulin use for type 2 diabetes, 2018-30: a microsimulation analysis. Lancet Diabetes Endocrinol 2019; 7(1):25–33.
14. Cho NH, Shaw JE, Karuranga S, et al. IDF Diabetes Atlas: Global estimates of diabetes prevalence for 2017 and projections for 2045. Diabetes Res Clin Pract 2018;138:271–81.
15. Prevention CfDCa. National Diabetes Statistics Report, 2017. Atlanta, GA 2017 2017.
16. Bullard KM, Cowie CC, Lessem SE, et al. Prevalence of diagnosed diabetes in adults by diabetes type - United States, 2016. MMWR Morb Mortal Wkly Rep 2018;67(12):359–61.
17. Nathan DM, Genuth S, Lachin J, et al. The effect of intensive treatment of diabetes on the development and progression of long-term complications in insulin-dependent diabetes mellitus. N Engl J Med 1993;329(14):977–86.

18. Nathan DM, Group DER. The diabetes control and complications trial/epidemiology of diabetes interventions and complications study at 30 years: overview. Diabetes care 2014;37(1):9–16.
19. Chiang JL, Kirkman MS, Laffel LMB, et al. Type 1 Diabetes Sourcebook A. Type 1 diabetes through the life span: a position statement of the American Diabetes Association. Diabetes care 2014;37(7):2034–54.
20. Standards of Medical Care in Diabetes-2019 Abridged for Primary Care Providers. Clin Diabetes 2019;37(1):11–34.
21. Walker AF, Hall JM, Shenkman B, et al. Geographic Access to Pediatrics Endocrinologists for Florida's publicly insured children with diabetes. Am J Manag Care 2018;24(4):106–9.
22. Klonoff DC. Using telemedicine to improve outcomes in diabetes–an emerging technology. J Diabetes Sci Technol 2009;3(4):624–8.
23. McDonnell ME. Telemedicine in complex diabetes management. Curr Diab Rep 2018;18(7):42.
24. Raymond JK, Berget CL, Driscoll KA, et al. CoYoT1 clinic: innovative telemedicine care model for young adults with type 1 diabetes. Diabetes Technol Ther 2016; 18(6):385–90.
25. Arora S, Geppert CM, Kalishman S, et al. Academic health center management of chronic diseases through knowledge networks: Project ECHO. Acad Med 2007;82(2):154–60.
26. Arora S, Kalishman S, Thornton K, et al. Expanding access to hepatitis C virus treatment–Extension for Community Healthcare Outcomes (ECHO) project: disruptive innovation in specialty care. Hepatology 2010;52(3):1124–33.
27. Arora S, Thornton K, Murata G, et al. Outcomes of treatment for hepatitis C virus infection by primary care providers. N Engl J Med 2011;364(23):2199–207.
28. ECHO Institate. Available at: https://echo.unm.edu/. Accessed May 21, 2021.
29. Bouchonville MF, Hager BW, Kirk JB, et al. Endo ECHO improves patient-reported measures of access to care, health care quality, self-care behaviors, and overall quality of life for patients with complex diabetes in medically underserved areas of New Mexico. Endocr Pract 2018;24(1):40–6.
30. Bouchonville MF, Paul MM, Billings J, et al. Taking telemedicine to the next level in diabetes population management: a review of the endo ECHO model. Curr Diab Rep 2016;16(10):96.
31. Cuttriss N, Anez-Zabala C, Baer LG, et al. 338-OR: leveraging the project ECHO model for Type 1 diabetes (T1D) in California and Florida: democratizing knowledge in underserved T1D communities. Diabetes 2019;68(Supplement 1): 338-OR.
32. Brink SJ, Miller M, Moltz KC. Education and multidisciplinary team care concepts for pediatric and adolescent diabetes mellitus. J Pediatr Endocrinol Metab 2002; 15(8):1113–30.
33. Wagner EH. The role of patient care teams in chronic disease management. BMJ 2000;320(7234):569–72.
34. Zurawski A, Komaromy M, Ceballos V, et al. Project ECHO brings innovation to community health worker training and support. J Health Care Poor Underserved 2016;27(4a):53–61.
35. Foster NC, Beck RW, Miller KM, et al. State of type 1 diabetes management and outcomes from the T1D exchange in 2016-2018. Diabetes Technol Ther 2019; 21(2):66–72.
36. Zhou C, Crawford A, Serhal E, et al. The impact of project ECHO on participant and patient outcomes: a systematic review. Acad Med 2016;91(10):1439–61.

37. Khunti S, Khunti K, Seidu S. Therapeutic inertia in type 2 diabetes: prevalence, causes, consequences and methods to overcome inertia. Ther Adv Endocrinol Metab 2019;10. 2042018819844694.

38. Rubino A, McQuay LJ, Gough SC, et al. Delayed initiation of subcutaneous insulin therapy after failure of oral glucose-lowering agents in patients with Type 2 diabetes: a population-based analysis in the UK. Diabet Med 2007;24(12):1412–8.

39. Russell-Jones D, Pouwer F, Khunti K. Identification of barriers to insulin therapy and approaches to overcoming them. Diabetes Obes Metab 2018;20(3):488–96.

40. Stanford ECHO Diabetes in the Time of COVID-19. Available at: http://diabetescovid.stanford.edu/. Accessed May 21, 2020.

Child Health and Telehealth in Global, Underresourced Settings

Julianna C. Hsing, BA[a,b,*], C. Jason Wang, MD, PhD[b,c],
Paul H. Wise, MD, MPH[b,c]

KEYWORDS

- Telehealth • Child health • Developing countries • Nutrition • Global

KEY POINTS

- Childhood mortality continues to be a public health priority worldwide.
- The application of telehealth to pediatric health care settings may be important to improving child health in developing countries.
- Despite barriers, pediatric telehealth has been used to improve health communication, assist clinical consultations, promote task-shifting, and support risk-shifting.
- Successful integration of telehealth to improve child health in developing countries may require an approach that is family-centered, culturally sustainable, and long-term developed.

INTRODUCTION

Telehealth, also known as telemedicine, is defined as the use of any form of information and communication technologies to exchange health information and provide health care services across geographic, time, social, cultural, and political barriers.[1] Over the years, telehealth (including mobile health [mHealth]) has been used to improve health care delivery in several ways, including improving access to health care, enhancing the quality of service delivery, improving the effectiveness of public health and primary care interventions, and improving the global shortage of health professionals through collaboration and training.[2]

Despite an increase in the number of published articles on the concept of telemedicine, many of these studies have taken place in industrialized countries. Few studies

[a] Department of Epidemiology and Population Health, Stanford University School of Medicine, 150 Governor's Lane, Stanford, CA 94305, USA; [b] Center for Policy, Outcomes and Prevention, Stanford University School of Medicine, 117 Encina Commons, Stanford, CA 94305, USA; [c] Department of Pediatrics, Stanford University School of Medicine, 291 Campus Drive, Stanford, CA 94305, USA
* Corresponding author. 117 Encina Commons, Stanford, CA 94305.
E-mail address: jchsing@stanford.edu

Pediatr Clin N Am 67 (2020) 773–781
https://doi.org/10.1016/j.pcl.2020.04.014
0031-3955/20/© 2020 Elsevier Inc. All rights reserved.
pediatric.theclinics.com

to date have reported the integration of telehealth within the pediatric health care system, especially in the context of the developing world, or low- and middle-income countries. A reason for this may be relative lack of rigorous research data to demonstrate that telehealth is indeed improving the delivery of pediatric health care. Such barriers as high costs, the lack of technical expertise, and the obstacle of establishing the necessary operational infrastructure are challenges in low-resource countries.[3] The growth of telehealth is opening new avenues for efficient, effective, and affordable pediatric health care services worldwide. However, a clearer understanding of the current landscape of pediatric telehealth in a global setting is strongly needed. To assess this landscape and its barriers, this article (1) provides examples of the current uses of pediatric telehealth in a global setting, (2) discusses key aspects of how telehealth can become successfully integrated in underresource countries, and (3) reviews the challenges that telehealth faces in said countries.

PEDIATRIC TELEHEALTH IN GLOBAL SETTINGS: AN OVERVIEW

Through our review of the literature, we found that telehealth has been used to: (1) improve health communication, (2) assist clinical consultations, (3) promote task-shifting, and (4) support risk-shifting in developing countries. To help illustrate these uses, we showcase examples from the literature of various health care programs worldwide, including one that was initiated by our faculty at Stanford University's Center for Health Policy.

Telehealth to Improve Health Communication: Stanford University's Guatemala Rural Child Health and Nutrition Program

With the evolution of the Internet and mobile phones from basic (voice only) to smartphones (text, voice, video, Internet, and gaming capabilities), it is natural that global health programs have leveraged telehealth technologies to support clinical practices by enhancing communication and improving care coordination for patients.[4–6] This has intuitive appeal, because many mHealth tools enable specialized physicians to provide health services far from the clinical setting, in remote areas, and among hard to reach communities.

Guatemala is one of the poorest countries and has one of the highest malnutrition rates in the world, with around 50% of all malnourished children in Central America residing in Guatemala.[7] To mitigate this, the Guatemala Rural Child Health and Nutrition Program was initiated to address the high rates of malnutrition, stunting, and child mortality in San Lucas Toliman, Guatemala. This program is a collaboration led by Dr Paul Wise and researchers at Stanford University and the larger system of community health promoters in Guatemala who are trained in a variety of areas, including hygiene, family education, nutrition supplementation, and primary medical care. Currently serving around 15,000 people in 22 communities, the Guatemala Rural Child Health and Nutrition Program has made a unique impact in the delivery of care in Mayan Guatemalan communities through the incorporation of an innovative mobile application (app) platform in the nutrition program. In working closely with the health promoters in Guatemala, Wise and his team designed an app that fit into their existing workflow, including the process of uploading patient data on the server via the dedicated Internet access point at the lead promoter's home. Routine follow-up care was much easier with the mobile app, because predictive algorithms were incorporated that immediately notified a health care promoter of when a child may soon fall to a more severe grade of malnutrition, and if intensive intervention will be warranted. In addition, the app automatically plotted the weight and height onto growth charts, relieving health promoters from the burden of hand-plotting data onto growth charts. Analysis of the pilot data from using the mobile app showed that training time for promoters was reduced from 3 years to less than 6 months, which has only positively contributed to the continual decrease in child mortality and stunting from severe malnutrition.

Using Telehealth Technologies to Assist Specialized Consultations in the Remote Clinic

Several telemedicine networks around the world deliver services to support children and families on a routine basis, many to low-income countries. Examples of these services include: acute-care visits at day care centers, pretransport assessment of critically ill children at community hospital, in-home remote monitoring, and subspecialty consultations (eg, cardiology, radiology, neurology, general surgery) that support primary care pediatricians in remote areas.[8–13]

- *Case 1: Children's National Medical Center: the pediatric telecardiology program*
  Live transmission of echocardiograms from remote sites to the Children's National Medical Center is one of the most commonly used applications among its many international telehealth programs.[14] Published reports of its use have shown that real-time guidance and immediate interpretation of echocardiograms is feasible and accurate, resulting in timely transport of critically ill children with heart disease and preventing unnecessary transport of children with normal hearts.[15] In addition to providing improvements to patient management, this method can also help local sonographic technicians perform higher quality echocardiograms. Since the program began in 1998, more than 6000 studies have been performed from 10 regional hospitals and several international partners, including Qatar, Morocco, Uganda, and Germany.[14] Today, live synchronous video transmission is used to address other medical problems, including those related to maternal and child health, malnutrition, and infectious disease prevention.
- *Case 2: Medical Missions for Children: the telemedicine outreach program*
  Medical Missions for Children (MMC) is a US nonprofit organization that operates a global videoconferencing network. It delivers expertise from medical specialists and technicians based in hospitals in the United States to children needing care in developing countries by using telemedicine.[16] The mission of MMC is to improve health care for children in medically underserved communities by using telemedicine.[16] Through its telemedicine outreach program, which is a distance medicine network that electronically connects physicians to patients in more than 100 remote countries, MMC partnered with the University Hospital in Brazil and donated two telemedicine units to this hospital so that they could have consultations with the tertiary care hospitals in the United States. Through this partnership, MMC has been able to facilitate teleconsultations for physicians and other local health professionals needing advice about clinical management for their patients, and also provide a valuable learning experience for all medical professionals involved in the process.[17]

Using Telehealth to Promote Task-Shifting from Physician to Community Health Workers

One of the main constraints in public health work is chronic shortage of well-trained health workers. Although this shortage is global, low- and middle-income countries, where such diseases as human immunodeficiency virus (HIV) and AIDS are a burden, feel this shortage the most. For instance, in Uganda, the shortage of health workers is so extreme that several districts have no physicians at all.[18] As a result, in 2006, the World Health Organization launched a task-shifting plan to strengthen and expand the pool of human resources for health. According to the World Health Organization, task-shifting is a process of delegation whereby tasks are moved, where appropriate, to less specialized health workers, and when combined with the tools used in telemedicine, the benefits are great.[18]

- *Case 1: Task-shifting in Uganda for HIV/AIDS antiretroviral therapy*
  In Uganda, task-shifting is currently the basis for providing antiretroviral therapy. Generally, providing antiretroviral therapy to 1000 individuals in settings in which resources are constrained requires an estimated one to two doctors, up to seven nurses, about three pharmacy staff, and a wide range of community workers. However, with only one doctor for every 22,000 patients and an overall health worker deficit of up to 80%, Uganda was forced to make task-shifting work. Nurses now undertake a range of tasks that were formerly the responsibility of doctors, whereas community health workers, who have training but not professional qualifications, are taking over tasks that were previously the responsibility of nurses. Examples of responsibilities that have been task-shifted to nurses include: managing coinfections in people with HIV, prescribing medication to prevent coinfection, determining clinical stage of people with HIV, and deciding eligibility for HIV therapy. Tasks that have been shifted to community health workers include: taking vital signs, HIV testing, counseling and education on antiretroviral therapy, monitoring and supporting adherence to therapy, and basic clinical follow-up.[19]

  However, having quality and supportive supervision and clinical mentoring when task-shifting antiretroviral therapy is important, especially in resource-constrained health settings where the health system is already weak and overwhelmed. Moreover, the complex referral process and subsequent consultation is still a frustrating challenge for patients and health care workers due to long waiting times, delays in and duplication of laboratory results, the cost of travel, and the time taken to consult a specialist.[20] Telemedicine can help address these problems by providing quality, clinical mentoring, timely access to a specialist, reducing the need and associated costs of travel, reductant consultation waiting times, and promoting home-based care.

- *Case 2: Task-shifting through community health promoters in Guatemala*
  A unique aspect of the nutrition program in Guatemala is the intentional task-shifting of roles from physicians to the community health promoters. They accomplish this by using a "train the trainer" approach where study staff and physicians provide extensive training locally and remotely to lead promoters. In turn, these lead promoters train other promoters and other trainees. As a result, community health promoters are not just focused on growth monitoring and providing supplements. Rather, they see their role as much larger where they can collectively work together to address larger community-level issues at hand. The promoter training curriculum also includes lessons on how to navigate and use the app, because they will eventually be the ones collecting data via the app's platform when Stanford physicians are not onsite.

Task-shifting expands the human resource pool rapidly and efficiently by building bridges among the health facility, its workers, the community, and patients.[18] When combined with telemedicine, training a new community health worker is completed in a much shorter period of time than it would usually take to train to be a licensed nurse. Task-shifting can also lead to the demographic reorganization of services and help them to move closer to the communities where they are needed. Local services provided by community health workers have been shown to bring positive benefits in an increased uptake of services, more timely detection and treatment, avoidance of overtreatment, and enhanced adherence to treatment.[18]

Use of Telehealth to Support Risk-Shifting in Developing Countries

Unstable governments and internal violence are common barriers in the developing world. However, telehealth can help overcome these barriers, because it is capable of putting specialized health care providers out of immediate risk. Telehealth can also offer the tools to provide support in response to disaster-based humanitarian need. Studies have shown that major medical and public health benefits can be provided even 3 to 6 months after disasters.[21]

- *Case 1: Delivering health services in areas of unstable governance and conflict through the Guatemala Rural Child Health and Nutrition Program*
  Rural areas, such as San Lucas Toliman, Guatemala, in developing countries are characterized by lack of resources and scarcity of communications infrastructure. These circumstances make it difficult to provide appropriate health care services. In Guatemala in particular, the 36-year-long civil war created a significant strain on health services and systems. However, innovative tools, such as telehealth, can be used for diagnosis and management to deliver patient care in underserved clinics and hospitals. Moreover, bringing external expertise through online consultation and the use of remote monitoring in areas of high demand may be valuable. Through the Guatemala nutrition initiative, Wise and his team at Stanford and other government officials have discussed efforts in discovering new technologies that can address the political barriers that exist in these areas. This is important so that in case of future internal conflicts, health care professionals and volunteer workers can take appropriate actions to protect themselves and reduce their risk of danger or being targeted.
- *Case 2: Telemedicine in the conflict, war-torn region of Somalia*
  Médecins Sans Frontières (MSF), also known as Doctors Without Borders, is an international, independent, medical humanitarian organization best known for its projects in conflict zones and countries affected by endemic diseases. In Somalia, MSF runs a district hospital supported by a limited number of Somali clinicians. Expatriate health care staff are no longer physically on site because they face high security risks because of kidnappings and direct threats to life. As a result, many Somali clinicians now have little opportunity for continuing education, poor technical knowledge, and lack of exposure to new medical developments. To address this, MSF introduced the new idea of telemedicine in Somalia, specifically implementing a real-time exchange of audiovisual information between the clinicians in Somalia and a specialist pediatrician in Nairobi. This exportation of expertise instead of experts to Somalia proved to be effective not only in pediatric care management, but also in pediatric outcomes and also showed to have added value to Somalian clinicians.[21] More than 85% of the Somalian clinicians surveyed noted that telemedicine was useful in helping to improve recognition of risk signs and to improve management protocols and prescription practices.[21] After sufficient training, all clinicians were eventually able to use the technology in an independent manner. Because they work under deprived and insecure circumstances in the world, Somalian doctors believed

strongly that telemedicine brought a sense of proximity and closeness with their tele-colleagues in Kenya.

- Case 3: The Haiti earthquake in 2010
  Investment in telemedicine capabilities has also the potential to reduce the over-all medical costs for deploying and supporting medical personnel to disaster areas. In many developing countries, such as Haiti, poor operational and communication infrastructure leaves thousands of individuals without access to basic health services. For instance, when an earthquake struck Haiti in 2010, the National Aeronautics and Space Administration was unable to support the victims of the earthquake because of the lack of resources and infrastructure.[22] Telephones, although vital for the coordination of relief efforts and for the dissemination of information to families, were poorly established.[23] Moreover, connectivity to Internet servers was almost nonexistent, and thus improvised. Satellites in Miami helped link a team in Florida to communicate requests for medical supplies and medications to specialist consultants. Physicians also used satellites for triage and video consultations, and because many patients had crush injuries, physicians on the ground in Haiti video conferenced with burn surgeons in Miami to discuss how best to treat the extremity wounds.[24]

Because many developing countries are areas where conflict or natural disasters makes it difficult to seek appropriate medical attention, telemedicine can help shift and reduce the risk for the health care professional by delivering care remotely.

INTEGRATING TELEHEALTH IN THE COMMUNITY CONTEXT OF RESOURCE-CONSTRAINED COUNTRIES

It is clear that developing countries have different health issues and needs than those of developed countries (eg, poverty, communicable diseases, maternal child health/infant mortality, workforce shortage, limited availability of broad-band Internet, high communication costs, low technological and educational literacy levels, language barriers).[1] What, then, allows certain telehealth programs to work in developing countries?

- Centering care around family and from within the community: The family unit is one of the most important aspects of many cultures. Therefore, it is important to consider telehealth as an enhancement to existing human and cultural relationships. This approach may be especially beneficial in pediatric health care settings, because care always involves the child and parent. In Guatemala, Wise and his team ensured that the foundation of the health promoters program was built on the family unit so that trust is established with the families they service. Moreover, the health promoters program empowers local community workers to play a larger role in the well-being of other community members through the "train the trainer" approach. Although the Stanford team has expert knowledge in implementing nutrition growth intervention in the area, they view community health workers as "key collaborators," who share insights for taking care of the local communities.
- Using appropriate and culturally acceptable technologies: Once the community has been understood, the appropriate technologies available are determined and become embedded into the local fabric of the community. This can become more apparent with the use of mobile phones for health-related concerns (eg, community announcements, appointment/check-up reminders) and with the

gathering of health volunteers and workers who meet regularly to attending training sessions. During the mobile app development project, Stanford researchers worked closely with many health promoters across 22 different Mayan communities to codesign a user interface that would be most useful for them and would make tracking nutrition faster, easier, and more accurate. Additionally, the hope of this codesign process was to lower the training requirements so that health promoters and the locals still support the service after the "foreign developer" (ie, Stanford) has left that area. Over time, the health workers slowly developed the confidence in the new skills they needed to learn to help others within the community.

- *Long-term collaboration and continuation of care:* By combining an mHealth approach with an established, 10-plus-year relationship among outside physicians, local clinicians, and the local health promoters of Guatemala, the nutrition program was not only able to increase the inflow of patients, but also provide seamless continuation of care. Health care promoters have taken over a large part of the role of routine follow-up care, health management, and coordinating with various nonprofits who offer assistance. It is important for future telehealth efforts to be put in the context of the critical health needs of Guatemala and to blend into its current and future health care system. Our hope is that through the Guatemala Rural Child Health and Nutrition Program and its efforts in using technological innovations, we can expand and enhance population health management, care coordination, and individualized care in the Highlands of Guatemala.

CURRENT CHALLENGES OF TELEMEDICINE IN A GLOBAL SETTING

Telehealth alters traditional concepts of what constitutes the patient-doctor relationship by imposing a physical distance between the doctor and its patient. Although it has been reported that most diagnoses can be made through history taking and with a proxy examination performed by the health worker in the room with the patient, the pivotal question remains: does telemedicine enhance or detract from the therapeutic relationship between doctor and patient?[25] Especially in certain cultures where family and community are highly valued, a modern concept like telemedicine may meet some resistance and can lead to compromises in the quality of care.[1,26,27] Moreover, the nuances of body language and nonverbal communication are frequently lost in telemedicine interactions. If the health care provider is too focused on the interpreter present in the room, which may draw the physician's attention away from the patient, he or she may miss important aspects of the patient's behavior that could impact the diagnosis. In cases when a family member serves as the interpreter, they may not understand certain medical terms being discussed, leading to important points getting lost in translation.

Currently, most telehealth programs in the developing world tend to narrowly focus on one disease (eg, telecardiology, teleradiology, telesurgery). However, the reality is that patients typically do not have "one disease," and those who do benefit from telesurgery or telecardiology are only a small fraction of the world's population. Therefore, solutions for the developing world need to be more pragmatic in addressing the specific needs and contexts of the developing world.

Although Internet connectivity and signal quality (eg, 2G to 3G to 4G) has improved dramatically over the years, it is inevitable for poorer, lower-resource areas to be left without connectivity because of their inability to have ready access and ability as quick as other developed areas. The lack of systems support and update may lead to higher levels of virus and worm infections of electronic patient data, potential breaches of security, or engagement of terrorist tactics to reach political ends. In addition to limited connectivity, resources to own a cell phone are not common, meaning may patients may share phones to receive messages from their health provider. However, with different health-related messages for different patients being sent to the same phone, they are bound to receive health-related messages for other people, which is a potential breach of personal health information.

SUMMARY

Telehealth has a unique position in the delivery of health care at a global setting. It can provide value, particularly when it is used in the right context to strengthen and support a local team. Although the place of telemedicine in direct patient care delivery remains to be established, currently it is important for training of local health care professionals. As technology availability and evidence-based telehealth models increase, it is hoped the barriers surrounding telehealth will begin to fall one by one. Until then, more high-quality, evidence-based studies on effectiveness and safety of pediatric telehealth practice are strongly needed, and the faster the trust relationships between remote doctors and physicians are established, the quicker telemedicine services can take hold in the relevant communities.

DISCLOSURE

The authors have nothing to disclose.

REFERENCES

1. Scott R, Mars M. Telehealth in the developing world: current status and future prospects. Smart Homecare Technol Telehealth 2015;25. https://doi.org/10.2147/shtt.s75184.
2. Ray Dorsey E, Topol EJ. State of telehealth. N Engl J Med 2016;375(2):154–61.
3. Olson CA, Mcswain SD, Curfman AL, et al. The current pediatric telehealth landscape. Pediatrics 2018;141(3). https://doi.org/10.1542/peds.2017-2334.
4. Piette JD, Datwani H, Gaudioso S, et al. Hypertension management using mobile technology and home blood pressure monitoring: results of a randomized trial in two low/middle-income countries. Telemed J E Health 2012;18(8):613–20.
5. Abdulrahman SA, Ganasegeran K. m-Health in public health practice: A Constellation of Current Evidence. In: Jude HD, Balas VE, editors. Telemedicine technologies: Big Data, Deep Learning, Robotics, Mobile and Remote Applications for Global Healthcare. Elsevier Inc; 2019. p. 171–82.
6. Ganasegeran K, Abdulrahman SA. Adopting m-Health in clinical practice: A Boon or a Bane?. In: Jude HD, Balas VE, editors. Telemedicine technologies: Big Data, Deep Learning, Robotics, Mobile and Remote Applications for Global Healthcare. Elsevier Inc; 2019. p. 31–41.
7. Chary A, Messmer S, Sorenson E, et al. The normalization of childhood disease: an ethnographic study of child malnutrition in rural Guatemala. Hum Organ 2013;72(2):87–97.
8. Satou GM, Rheuban K, Alverson D, et al. Telemedicine in pediatric cardiology: a scientific statement from the American Heart Association. Circulation 2017;135. https://doi.org/10.1161/CIR.0000000000000478.
9. Kuhle S, Mitchell L, Andrew M, et al. Urgent clinical challenges in children with ischemic stroke: analysis of 1065 patients from the 1-800-NOCLOTS pediatric stroke telephone consultation service. Stroke 2006;37(1):116–22.

10. Otero AV, Lopez-Magallon AJ, Jaimes D, et al. International telemedicine in pediatric cardiac critical care: a multicenter experience. Telemed J E Health 2014; 20(7):619–25.

11. Heath B, Salerno R, Hopkins A, et al. Pediatric critical care telemedicine in rural underserved emergency departments. Pediatr Crit Care Med 2009;10(5):588–91.

12. McConnochie KM, Wood NE, Kitzman HJ, et al. Telemedicine reduces absence resulting from illness in urban child care: evaluation of an innovation. Pediatrics 2005;115(5):1273–82.

13. Mahnke CB, Jordan CP, Bergvall E, et al. The Pacific asynchronous teleHealth (PATH) system: review of 1,000 pediatric teleconsultations. Telemed J E Health 2011;17(1):35–9.

14. Alverson DC, Swinfen LR, Swinfen LP, et al. Transforming systems of care for children in the global community efforts should be aimed at improving. Pediatr Ann 2009;579–86. https://doi.org/10.3928/00904481-20090918.

15. Sable C, Roca T, Gold J, et al. Live transmission of neonatal echocardiograms from underserved areas: accuracy, patient care, and cost. Telemed J 1999; 5(4):339–47.

16. Children MM for. Global medicine and teaching networks. Available at: www.mmis-sions.org/index.html. Accessed August 29, 2019.

17. Ozuah PO, Renzik M. Medical Missions for Children: a global telemedicine and teaching network. In: Wootton R, Patil NG, Scott RE, et al, editors. Telehealth in the developing world. Royal Society of Medicine Press Ltd; International Development Research Centre; 2009. p. 101–8.

18. World Health Organization. Taking stock task shifting to tackle health worker shortages.; 2007.

19. Baine SO, Kasangaki A. A scoping study on task shifting: the case of Uganda. BMC Health Serv Res 2014;14(1):1–11.

20. Kiberu VM, Scott RE, Mars M. Assessing core, e-learning, clinical and technology readiness to integrate telemedicine at public health facilities in Uganda: a health facility-based survey. BMC Health Serv Res 2019;19(1):1–11.

21. Zachariah R, Bienvenue B, Ayada L, et al. Practicing medicine without borders: tele-consultations and tele-mentoring for improving paediatric care in a conflict setting in Somalia? Trop Med Int Health 2012;17(9):1156–62.

22. Nicogossian AE, Doarn CR. Armenia 1988 earthquake and telemedicine: lessons learned and forgotten. Telemed J E Health 2011;17(9):741–5.

23. Brauman R. Haiti earthquake: what priorities? Centre de Reflexion sur l'Action et les Savoirs Humanitaires (CRASH) Foundation Medecins Sans Frontieres. 2010. Available at: https://www.msf-crash.org/en/publications/natural-disasters/haiti-earthquake-what-priorities. Accessed September 6, 2019.

24. Louden K. Telemedicine connects earthquake-ravaged Haiti to the world 2010. Available at: https://www.medscape.com/viewarticle/717232. Accessed September 6, 2019.

25. Wootton R, Darkins A. Telemedicine and the doctor-patient relationship. J R Coll Physicians Lond 1997;31(6):6–7.

26. Gogia SB, Maeder A, Mars M, et al. Unintended consequences of tele health and their possible solutions. Contribution of the IMIA Working Group on Telehealth. Yearb Med Inform 2016. https://doi.org/10.15265/IY-2016-012.

27. Institute of Medicine. The role of telehealth in an evolving health care environment: workshop summary. Washington, DC: The National Academies Press; 2012.

Moving?

Make sure your subscription moves with you!

To notify us of your new address, find your **Clinics Account Number** (located on your mailing label above your name), and contact customer service at:

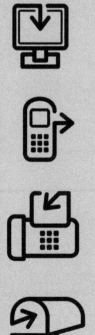

Email: journalscustomerservice-usa@elsevier.com

800-654-2452 (subscribers in the U.S. & Canada)
314-447-8871 (subscribers outside of the U.S. & Canada)

Fax number: 314-447-8029

Elsevier Health Sciences Division
Subscription Customer Service
3251 Riverport Lane
Maryland Heights, MO 63043

*To ensure uninterrupted delivery of your subscription, please notify us at least 4 weeks in advance of move.

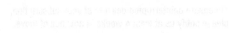

Printed and bound by CPI Group (UK) Ltd, Croydon, CR0 4YY

03/10/2024

01040401-0018